MILLIONS OF AMERICANS HAVE DIFFICULTY UNDERSTANDING SPOKEN LANGUAGE.

THEY'RE NOT DEAF, AUTISTIC, OR SLOW. THEY HAVE APD.

APD has been called the auditory equivalent of dyslexia, and its debilitating effects cross all ages, genders, and races. APD can cause children to fail in school and adults to suffer socially and in their careers, but until now, there has been little information available.

Written by Dr. Teri James Bellis, one of the world's foremost authorities on APD, this is the first book on the subject that is completely accessible to the public. *When the Brain Can't Hear* gives you all the latest information:

- What is APD?
- How APD affects children
- APD in adults
- Diagnosis and testing
- Treatment options
- Living successfully with APD
- Memory enhancement and other coping techniques

WHEN THE BRAIN CAN'T HEAR

UNRAVELING THE MYSTERY OF
AUDITORY PROCESSING DISORDER

Teri James Bellis, Ph.D.

ATRIA BOOKS
NEW YORK LONDON TORONTO SYDNEY

ATRIA BOOKS
1230 Avenue of the Americas
New York, NY 10020

ISBN: 0-7434-2863-3
     0-7434-2864-1 (Pbk)

First Atria Books trade paperback edition July 2003

10 9 8 7 6

ATRIA BOOKS is a trademark of Simon & Schuster, Inc.

Manufactured in the United States of America

For information regarding special discounts for bulk purchases,
please contact Simon & Schuster Special Sales at 1-800-456-6798 or
business@simonandschuster.com

ACKNOWLEDGMENTS

IN SPORTS, THERE ARE halls of fame that recognize those players who have contributed the most, scored the greatest number of points, and changed the course of history through their effort, talent, knowledge, and sheer determination. If there were a hall of fame to honor the professionals and scientists who have shaped our current conceptualization of auditory processing disorders (APD), the walls would be lined with names such as Gail Chermak, Jeanane Ferre, Jack Katz, Robert Keith, James Jerger, Frank Musiek, Jack Willeford, and many more. These are the people who have laid the stones on the circuitous path toward unraveling the mystery of what happens when the brain can't "hear." I am indebted to their years of contribution and dedication to the field, and this book could never have been written without them.

Of these, three in particular have been invaluable to me both personally and professionally, and I am proud to call them colleagues and friends. Without question, Dr. Frank Musiek, Director of Audiology and Professor of Otolaryngology and Neurology at the Dartmouth-Hitchcock Medical Center in Lebanon, New Hampshire, has contributed more to our understanding of how lesions or dysfunction in specific brain regions affect auditory processing than anyone else in the field. He has also had the greatest influence on me, personally, by taking me under his wing several years ago and filling my brain with all of the basic knowledge upon which I have built in the years since. To this day, Frank remains a valued friend and mentor. There is no doubt in my mind that, if not for him, I would not be where I am now, doing something I love so much. He was the first to believe in me, and I hope my subsequent work has proven me worthy of that belief.

We owe our current knowledge of how higher-order metacognitive and metalinguistic factors affect auditory processing largely to the efforts of Dr. Gail Chermak, Distinguished Professor of Audiology and Chair of the Department of Speech and Hearing Sciences at Washington State University, Pullman. Her work has made all of us look at information (especially spoken language) processing in its entirety and acknowledge the need to consider both bottom-up and top-down factors in assessing and managing APD. Personally, Gail has done far more than she realizes to make me feel welcome in this field. She is always approachable and supportive, never ego-bound, and is such an engaging speaker that I could listen to her for hours without a hint of boredom. As a role model, Gail represents a standard of personal and professional integrity and accomplishment to which I can only hope to aspire.

Last, but certainly not least, is my "partner in crime," Dr. Jeanane Ferre of Oak Park, Illinois, without whom, frankly, there would be no Bellis/Ferre model of APD. As one of the only professionals in the country, whose private practice consists solely of assessment and management of APD, she has done much to further our understanding of the relationship between auditory processing and language, learning, and communication. A close friend as well as a colleague, Jeanane has always been there to help me through the crises and applaud my successes. She also happens to be the only person who can put up with rooming with me at national conventions, which says a lot about her personally. Jeanane likes to say that she and I are of such like minds that we share one brain. I thank her for letting me use it during the writing of this book and promise to return it to her when I am finished.

So many others have assisted me in countless ways that I cannot possibly mention them all. I would, however, like to thank my agent,

Jodie Rhodes, for taking a fledgling idea that I had been considering for years and guiding it to a level of fruition that I could never have dreamed possible; Tracy Behar, my editor at Pocket Books, who recognized the importance of this topic and trusted me to address it adequately; Brenda Copeland, associate editor at Pocket Books, who had the day-to-day task of trudging through pages and pages of drafts and E-mails and who always managed to make editorial suggestions that were not only insightful and improved my writing immeasurably, but were gently couched so as not to bruise the author's delicate ego; and Renee O'Connor and Tracy Olinger, both of whom read initial draft chapters and made valuable suggestions for strengthening them.

I am also grateful to my students and fellow faculty and staff members in the Department of Communication Disorders at the University of South Dakota, who never once complained during the frantic months when I was trying to fulfill my full-time obligation to them, write this book, and keep my sanity all at the same time. Instead, they were always ready with words of support and shoulders to lean on when the wild, panicked look in my eyes became frighteningly apparent.

For always reminding me of why I do what I do, I thank all of my patients—adults and children—with APD and their parents and loved ones. Their letters of gratitude, support, and encouragement mean more to me than any amount of professional success. I especially thank Jayna Newell and her son, Benjamin, who traveled across the country just to have lunch with me and share their story of frustration and, most importantly, success in coping with APD.

Finally, this book is dedicated to those who suffered the most during the writing of it: my husband, Tim, who read every word I wrote, compiled glossary terms, performed secretarial duties, cooked, cleaned, did the laundry, shuttled the kids from place to place, endured stress attacks and wild mood swings (mine, not his), yet still found the energy to say "I love you" at the end of every day; my daughter, Jennie, who had to entertain and watch over her brothers for months on end; and my sons, Chris and Danny, who heard the words "Don't bother Mommy, she's working right now" far more often than any little boys should ever have to hear. Always, they are the light that beckons to me from the end of the tunnel and the wind at my back that speeds me along.

CONTENTS

WALKING A MILE IN THEIR SHOES

I HAVE A BULLETIN board on the wall across from my desk. On it is a letter I received from the mother of a child with an auditory processing disorder (APD). For most of his young life, Jonathan had struggled with listening, learning, and communicating. Like a child with a hearing loss, Jonathan often had difficulty hearing what was being said, especially if there was a lot of noise around him. He couldn't tell the difference between certain speech sounds or connect them with the appropriate letters of the alphabet, so he couldn't read or write well. He had a hard time following directions and understanding information in school. Until quite recently, I had never actually met Jonathan face-to-face. But I felt as if I knew him well. His mother, Jane, and I had been in communication off and on for several years. I had reviewed Jonathan's records and test results and had made suggestions for treating his APD, educating his teachers about the disorder, and coping with the disorder at home. Jane's most recent letter to me, the one that is on my bulletin board, reads:

> Dear Dr. Bellis:
>
> I have an update with lots and lots of good news. Jonathan was chosen from his school as the first place winner in the science project (210 3rd graders). He has climbed to 4 A's and is about to get a B in writing, enough to qualify him for honor roll. Today he came home and his teacher's note was about a chapter book he had read and taken a test on. He made 100% on the test at a 3.8 reading level. Actually, a

little above where he is supposed to be! Just thought you should hear
the good news, since you've been in the trenches with me for so long.
Keep in touch. I know one of these days this case will be the one with
the happy ending.

Thanks,

Jane

I keep this letter on my bulletin board as a daily reminder that, when I talk or write about APD, I am talking and writing about real people: children and adults with names and faces. Girls and boys, men and women, all of whom have family members who love and worry about them. Real people who are struggling every day with all of the difficulties that can result from APD. And, when I sit down at my desk and see that letter, I am also reminded that, when APD is diagnosed and treated appropriately, there can be an end to—or at least a lessening of—their struggles. There can be a happy ending.

I am an audiologist—a specialist in hearing and its disorders. I am also a college professor, a wife, and a mother of three.

I have an auditory processing disorder.

Aha! You are probably thinking, "That must be why she became a specialist in auditory processing disorders."

Nope.

As a matter of fact, I didn't even know that I had an APD until long after I was entrenched in the field and had already published a textbook on the subject. Like most people, I seem to be good at figuring out what's going on with others, but poor at recognizing the same issues in myself.

Actually, my growing up with a deaf brother first sparked my interest in hearing. My intimate knowledge and understanding of the impact hearing disorders can have on learning and family life led me to major in deaf education in college. When I took my first introduction to audiology course, I became fascinated with the field of audiology, and that prompted me to change my major in my junior year. Finally, my first neuroanatomy class truly fired me up about this wonderful, fascinating, frustrating, enigmatic organ we call the brain. That's what led me to specialize in brain-based auditory disorders.

So, in an ironic twist of fate, I was a specialist in brain-related auditory disorders long before I myself became the victim of a brain-based auditory disorder as the result of an auto accident. And several years passed after that before I even had a clue about my own APD, despite my working with individuals with APD every day.

It took so long for me to recognize an APD in myself because, first, I don't conform to the "classic" picture of APD. Most individuals with APD have difficulty hearing in noise—I don't. Most individuals with APD frequently ask for repetitions—I don't. Most individuals with APD have difficulty comprehending or remembering complex verbal information—I don't. Most individuals with APD have greater difficulty in language- or auditory-based activities such as reading, spelling, writing, and speaking and fare far better in those areas that do not rely on auditory-language skills such as mathematics and art—I don't. Instead, I have always been an excellent reader and speller, and I can best express myself in writing, even today. On the other hand, I can't do math and my art skills are, shall we say, nonexistent.

My APD was merely one portion of a far greater constellation of symptoms resulting from my accident, most of which were far more obvious and disruptive to my life than the auditory component, at least in the years immediately following my head trauma. For example, in addition to the inevitable physical injuries and emotional trauma, I found that I had completely lost the ability to perform even the simplest of math calculations. Furthermore, my visual perceptual abilities were affected so severely that I couldn't perform even the most mundane of chores, such as shopping for groceries. I could not find even a single item I was looking for among the many similar items on the grocery store shelf. Indeed, visually complex environments made me so confused and dizzy that I just began avoiding them.

Moreover, I had lost what little art ability I'd once had. Whereas, once upon a time, I could draw a dog that bore at least some resemblance to man's best friend, now my dogs looked like a curious cross between a chicken and a forklift. Even my motor skills were affected: I suffered from partial paralysis and extremely poor coordination in my left arm and hand to the point that just holding a coffee cup became a chore requiring the utmost concentration and effort. Also disconcerting were my frequent experiences of déjà vu, something I had noticed on occasion throughout my life but that now seemed to occur with disturbing regularity and frequency.

I didn't seem to have any auditory difficulties whatsoever. I did begin to notice, however, that everyone from my husband to the clerk behind the checkout counter at the drugstore seemed to be speaking rather nastily to me. It wasn't so much *what* they said, but rather *how* they said it—depending on the situation, the tone of voice seemed either condescending, sarcastic, or just plain mean. I became convinced that everyone hated me, that they all had it in for me, else why would they speak to me so?

The doctors—and there were many—all put this last phenomenon down to "increased emotional lability following significant physical and emotional trauma." In layman's terms, I had been through a lot and I was, quite understandably, a little touchy. I couldn't make the doctors understand that the problem wasn't *my* emotional lability, but everyone else's inexcusable rudeness.

For two years I underwent batteries of tests designed to quantify and qualify the many difficulties I was having. The results were discouraging. Cognitive testing, for example, was a complete downer. Although I had once exhibited a Mensa-level IQ (I had skipped a grade as a child and, even then, was placed in special classrooms for gifted students), my new testing indicated an overall IQ in the low average range. I shouldn't have been surprised. Many of the IQ subtests rely on motor coordination, visual-perceptual skills, sequencing, memory, and the like—all the areas with which I was experiencing difficulty.

But still, dropping overnight from genius to average was a blow to my ego and an uncomfortable confirmation of just how much function I had lost.

Magnetic resonance imaging (MRI) and computerized tomography (CT) scans of my brain revealed little except for some slight swelling around my brain stem and upper cervical region, as well as an almost imperceptible swelling around the right temporal lobe of my brain that went away relatively quickly. Many of my physical symptoms—neck and shoulder pain, severe headaches, dizziness—were probably related to this swelling. However, the MRI and CT testing shed little light on the reasons for my more subjective complaints of visual-spatial, mathematical, and art difficulties. Nor did they help me understand why, at this most difficult point in my life, everyone was talking to me in tones that suggested I was a child or an idiot or was loading each word with such dripping sarcasm or hostility that I had no option but to respond in kind.

I was miserable.

So, I suspect, was everyone who had to put up with me. I would cry at the drop of a hat. I would react defensively to even the slightest of perceived insults—whether real or imaginary. Because it seemed to me as though everyone was addressing me in an offensive tone of voice, I began to react defensively. Feelings were constantly hurt—my own and those of everyone around me.

Illumination of at least some of my subjective difficulties came completely inadvertently. I was assisting an intern under my supervision in learning the proper placement of scalp electrodes during auditory electrophysiologic testing. In this type of testing, sounds are delivered to the ear, and the brain's responses to these sounds are recorded. I, of course, had offered myself as the honorary guinea pig, as any good supervisor and scientist would. As I was describing the printout of results and how to interpret them, I realized that we had obtained only a small recorded response from the electrode placed over the right side of my head—one much smaller than that obtained over the left side of my head. Suspecting some type of equipment failure, we verified that all components were working fine, then repeated the testing. To our surprise, we got the same results—a definitive, clear sign of a neurophysiologic abnormality in or near the right temporal lobe of my brain.

These findings made me wonder how I would perform on the behavioral tests of auditory processing that I used with my patients, so I had my intern run me through all of them. We found that I had extreme difficulty with every task that relied on the right hemisphere of the brain. I couldn't discriminate between short tones that differed subtly in duration or pitch. I couldn't report words, numbers, or sentences that were delivered to my left ear when different stimuli were being delivered to my right ear simultaneously—a condition known as *dichotic listening.*

Subsequently, I consulted with a neuropsychiatrist who was trained in brain-behavior organization and was adept at synthesizing a variety of information from various disciplines. He confirmed what I had already begun to suspect: I was experiencing all the signs and symptoms of right-hemisphere dysfunction. My left-sided motor-control issues, visual-spatial difficulties, inability to perform mathematics, and similar complaints all supported such a diagnosis. Even my frequent feelings of déjà vu proved to be a common complaint following right-hemisphere, particularly temporal lobe, damage. Had I been a child, I might well have qualified for special education services under the label of "nonverbal—or right-hemisphere—learning disability," for I exhibited virtually all of the diagnostic indicators of this disorder.

Finally, my difficulty in perceiving the intent of others' communications was not simply a manifestation of increased emotionality. I was experiencing a fundamental inability to perceive subtle nonlinguistic aspects of the message, particularly related to tone of voice, that are important in determining what a person *means* in relation to what he or she *says*—a task that relies on the right hemisphere of the brain. I, the specialist in APD, had ended up with an APD myself.

To some degree, I felt vindicated when I received all this information. Now, I could prove that it wasn't all in my head. Instead, there were real, physiologically distinct reasons for my subjective complaints.

I felt vindicated, but I was not relieved. I could now understand on an intellectual level why I was experiencing the myriad difficulties that had plagued me since the accident, but this knowledge didn't seem to make me feel any better.

Actually, my reaction was quite typical when one considers the psychological and emotional stages of grief that are to be expected following the diagnosis of a disability. Because my symptoms were so obvious, I don't remember ever having experienced denial. Instead, my first reaction was anger, and my second was fear. Fear of the unknown. Fear of what would happen if I never improved in any of these areas. Fear of living with disability—something I had helped many patients to do, but never expected to have to deal with myself. And finally, fear that, as one of my early physicians had actually told me, I would never learn again, never really work again, never be able to return to school as I had always planned to obtain my doctorate.

Then came depression—quite common following trauma and a frequent occurrence in right-hemisphere disorders. Within a matter of months, my weight had dropped to double digits. I was unable to work or even to care for my child. All I could see were the walls of the bottomless pit I had plunged into. No light shining in from above. No ground below me. Just endless, infinite black.

It's been a long, hard journey. But in the years since my accident, I've learned how to put into practice the principles of good management that are appropriate not just for my disorder but for many other types of disability. I underwent cognitive retraining for my visual difficulties and physical therapy for my motor deficits, and although I still have some residual dysfunction, it's not all that apparent to anyone who isn't aware of it. I took time to consider realistic life choices, and I found new ways of performing in my chosen career.

One of the most difficult decisions I had to face was the need to change job settings. Before the accident, I was an audiologist who specialized in electrophysiologic techniques, even monitoring brain and nerve function during neurosurgery. But after the accident, I found that I could no longer perform my job competently. Even after therapy, my visual problems were so severe that I was unable to interpret rapidly and accurately what I was seeing on the computer screen during surgical procedures.

So I moved on to audiology in the school setting. Although leaving intraoperative monitoring behind was painful, even devastating, at the time, it turned out to be a blessing. For the first time in my career, my interest in brain function and pediatric audiology began to come together.

Gradually, these interests evolved into a new specialty area for me: APD. In the years since, I have evaluated and treated hundreds of children and adults with APD and have written a textbook designed to help other professionals in my own and related fields do the same. I have even put myself through my own auditory therapy techniques so that, now, I can at least discriminate subtle differences in pitch and I am quite a bit better at interpreting tone-of-voice cues from other people.

Eventually—and against all predictions made by my austere medical team in the years immediately following my accident—I was able even to return to school. I earned my doctorate from Northwestern University in Audiology and Hearing Sciences with a special emphasis in language and cognition—something that I accomplished, I am proud to say, in record time and with straight A's. I am teaching, writing, and lecturing in the areas of audiology and auditory processing now, and my students know that if I'm explaining a scientific concept that involves any mathematics, I will rely on them to do the addition and multiplication while I write on the board. In fact, in some strange way, some of my disabilities have evolved over the years into eccentricities that make me who I am today. I guess I've reached that final stage of grief: acceptance.

Still, it is the auditory deficit—subtle as it may be—that continues to be the most disruptive of my difficulties. I have to remind myself not to take it personally if a colleague or a friend seems abrupt or short or even angry at me. Although this would surprise many people who know me, I sometimes spend hours agonizing over possible hidden meanings that might be buried in day-to-day communications with my friends, family, and coworkers. Because I know that my perceptions may not always be representative of reality, I try not to respond from the gut when I feel that I am being attacked or put upon or patronized. It has taken me a long time, but I am finally beginning to enjoy social and professional success again.

On the other hand, I am not quite as careful a communicator at home. As a parent, I find myself endlessly uttering that time-honored command that I swore I would never subject my children to. You know the one: "Don't speak to me in that tone of voice!" There are, of course, occasions when those words are appropriate. However, I say them much more frequently than is warranted, often earning hurt looks of bewilderment and a deep, inner twinge of guilt for my behavior.

My husband was a huge factor in my recovery. As everyone is always telling me, much to my consternation at times, he is a wonderful fellow. And he could appreciate some of what I was experiencing as he had been involved in the same accident. But apparently because he had been in the rear passenger seat whereas I had been driving, his head bibbled when mine bobbled, and he ended up with more garden-variety injuries: neck and back pain, dizziness, headaches. I'm not saying he didn't suffer, but his brain, his remarkable artistic talent, his ability to think, all the factors that made up the essence of *him,* remained essentially unchanged after the accident. And, because I was an audiologist who frequently worked with post-head-trauma victims, his difficulties made fundamental, scientific sense to me. They were quantifiable. They were identifiable. They showed up on tests of balance function. They were what I was used to seeing every day in my hospital-based clinic.

That is, with one ironic exception.

In complete contrast to me, Tim had always been a visual learner. He is a talented artist, excellent at mazes and puzzles and dominoes, good at math. He excels at all of the activities that do nothing but frustrate me. Shortly after the accident, however, we began to notice that he was having difficulty hearing me, especially if the television was on too loud or water was running nearby. It wasn't very obvious at first, just occasional situations here and there in which he had a hard time understanding what I was saying. But, as the years went by, the problem became worse. Audiologic testing showed that his actual hearing acuity was normal, confirming that he didn't have a hearing loss that could account for his listening difficulties. Rather, it seemed as though he was merely becoming a typical, frustrating husband who, at some point in his midthirties or early forties, begins to tune out his wife. I had heard complaints from hundreds of women during my career about just such a tendency in their own husbands. Apparently, wonderful as he may be, my own husband was, at least in this respect, just like all the others.

In that, at least, I was right. Where I erred was in concluding that nothing physiologic was causing his hearing difficulty, that he was merely "tuning me out." As my own research would soon reveal, some men begin to exhibit auditory processing problems as a result of normal aging by about the age of thirty-five. Indeed, the common complaint of wives that their husbands seem not to listen anymore may well be due, at least in part, to adult-onset APD in men.

So we're quite a pair, Tim and I, he with his difficulty hearing in noise and me with my difficulty comprehending intent. At times, we find ourselves arguing ferociously over something I didn't say or something he didn't mean, a situation that would no doubt amuse the objective observer. Luckily, we have just enough understanding of and tolerance for the other's auditory deficit not to allow these occasional misunderstandings to drive a permanent wedge between us. Still, I can't help but wonder what life would be like without these difficulties.

Our problems are mild. Countless children and adults have much more significant and severe auditory processing deficits. The impact of these deficits on the lives of these people are often far-reaching and dramatic, affecting learning, language, socialization, and general life skills. As my own story demonstrates, auditory processing deficits can occur later in life, can result from factors such as trauma and aging, and can coexist with a host of other, seemingly unrelated, difficulties. So, too, can auditory processing deficits manifest themselves in early childhood, leading to difficulties in school, at home, and with friends. When dealing with APD, no two people are alike, and the impact of a deficit on one person's life may be quite different from the impact of the same deficit on another's. This heterogeneity leads to difficulties in defining, diagnosing, and treating these deficits. APD may be viewed as a beast with many faces, each of which presents a different picture to the world. Only by examining each of these faces can we hope to, finally, understand, and, yes, even accept this troublesome beast.

In my years of working with and studying APD and its impact on language, learning, and life in my patients and their families, one need has been articulated more often than any other. Without exception, each of the people with whom I have worked has expressed the need for information, tips, anything that can help to shed light on APD. They plead for resources that will assist in understanding and triumphing over the disorder. Or, if absolute triumph is not in the cards, they ask for guidance to help them learn to live successfully with the disorder. Many of the people who have been affected in some way by APD in their lives have expressed the wish for a book written specifically for them, in their language, to help them comprehend this most complex of subjects.

This is my gift to all those seeking such illumination. It comes from someone who understands what it is like to live with an APD. And it comes from someone who has spent the last several years trying to define and battle this beast, who has shared in the joy of successes and who has provided a shoulder upon which to weep when the barriers seemed too high to climb. It comes from the heart. And I hope, I dearly hope, that it provides some ray of light—however small, however dim—in the darkness.

THE MANY FACES OF APD

JEFF WAS SEVENTEEN years old, over six feet tall, and outweighed me by at least a hundred pounds. He was a big kid. Tough, too. He was one of the starring offensive linemen on his high school football team. Word had it that he could cut through the other team's defense like a knife through butter, scattering smaller players in all directions.

Yet, despite all of his toughness, he had a gentle, polite manner and a heart of gold. When Jeff and his mother arrived at the clinic, he greeted me with a shy smile. He was extremely cooperative during testing and apologized whenever he made a mistake or missed an item. He even called me "ma'am." I'm not too fond of that generally, but, coming from him, I found it quite endearing. Which is probably why I felt as if my heart were breaking when, halfway through my explanation of his test results, he dropped his head onto his folded hands and began to cry.

My voice stuttered to a stop. I laid my hand lightly on Jeff's shoulder, and he grasped it in his large, meaty palm and squeezed.

In a choked voice, he whispered, "I thought I was just stupid."

"What do you mean?"

He lifted his head and met my gaze. There was relief in his eyes, but also anger, embarrassment, and just a little defiance.

"You know, dumb jock. I just always figured I was stupid. That's why I couldn't get it. I was just a big, dumb jock. A joke."

These were astounding words coming from a boy who had just been elected "most popular" in his junior class and was a sure bet for prom king in his senior year.

Jeff had experienced academic difficulties ever since he had begun school. He had had problems learning to spell and read and still struggled with those subjects in his junior year in high school. He liked the idea of losing himself in a book, of journeying to far-off lands or reading about historical people, but he rarely opened a book unless forced to. Jeff had a difficult time sounding out the words, so his reading was slow and laborious. As he described it, by the time he figured out what the words were, he had lost the thread of the story.

But Jeff loved to spin tales. He would make up stories about princes and dragons, life in the circus and travels to outer space, and tell them to his younger brother, who would sit spellbound in wonder as the stories unfolded. Creative as he was, Jeff never wrote his stories down. As with his reading, spelling was a struggle, so much so that even if he focused on telling the story and just coming close enough to the spelling of the words so that he could return and correct them later, he was unable to understand his own writing when it came time to polish what he had set to paper. As a result, his English composition and creative writing papers were short, poorly organized, and contained only simple language and elementary vocabulary. They exhibited no hint whatsoever of the imaginative mind of the boy who held the pen.

Jeff came from a rural school district, and special education services were scarce. Nevertheless, during his elementary school years, he did qualify for reading remediation and tutoring under the classification of learning disability. Since junior high school, however, he had not received any services, primarily because he consistently earned A's and B's in all of his classes. Therefore, the school-based special education team had decided that his reading problems were no longer affecting him academically.

The reason for Jeff's apparent educational success was, unfortunately, all too common. As a student who excelled at football in a town where football was all-important, he had been passed through every class since he was in the ninth grade. No academic probation or C's for our boy, no, sir. In fact, his good academic record, combined with his amazing sports ability, had already resulted in offers of full-ride sports scholarships from several major universities—before he had even begun his senior year in high school.

Any other kid in his shoes would have been turning cartwheels.

But Jeff was different. He was acutely aware that he hadn't earned the grades he had been given. In fact, despite putting several hours into his studies every night after football practice, he knew that he should, by rights, barely be passing subjects such as social studies, history, and English composition.

His mother had initiated Jeff's referral to me for central auditory processing evaluation. Because she saw Jeff still struggling so hard with reading, she had arranged for independent, private testing by a specialist in learning disabilities. This testing had confirmed that Jeff exhibited low average to borderline abilities in reading decoding (e.g., sounding out words, or word-attack skills), general fund of knowledge, and auditory discrimination abilities. Other symptoms leading to the suspicion of auditory processing deficit were his difficulty following information presented in lectures and, particularly illuminating, his inability to hear the quarterback of his football team call plays during the huddle. "I can't ever hear him," he told me. "But I don't let on. I just keep my eye on where the ball is. I know what I'm supposed to do, so I just go out there and do it." In this manner, Jeff had succeeded in football without anyone being aware of what he had secretly come to call his "hearing problem."

In social situations, he frequently smiled his shy smile and nodded rather than jumping into the conversation, furthering others' perception of him as the sweet, strong, silent type. And when he was unable to answer questions posed directly to him or answered as if he hadn't been paying attention, he took the ribbing of his friends—still with the same, shy smile.

But inside Jeff was hurting.

"You're not stupid, Jeff," I told him. "You never were. You have what we call an auditory processing disorder. Basically, what this means is that your hearing itself is fine, but what gets into the ear somehow gets jumbled by the time it gets to the brain. Because of this, different letters may sound the same to you, making it hard to tell the difference between different speech sounds. Or you might hear what someone is saying, but it's distorted or muffled, like the person is mumbling, especially if there's a lot of noise around. If you can't hear the speech sounds clearly, it's hard to learn how to sound out words when you're reading or to spell them when you're writing. That's why you have to work so hard." With that, Jeff released my hand, nodded once, and listened while I explained the rest of the test results and what I thought we should do to help him overcome his disorder. A disorder that had a name for the first time. One that could be addressed, confronted, and although maybe not completely fixed, one for which he could at least learn ways of compensating.

That was when Jeff shared his dreams for the future with me. It wasn't enough for him to be popular, to be a football star, and to have a college education virtually handed to him on a platter. It wasn't enough that there was already talk of his possibly not needing to finish college, of being picked up by a farm team or even a pro team before he even reached his senior year at whatever university he chose.

Jeff had bigger plans. "I'm happy about the whole scholarship thing, sure," he admitted. "I mean, that'll get me there, pay for everything. And I like football. It's fun." He shrugged. "But I really want to do well in college. I want to *learn*. I don't want to be a football player for real, not after college. I mean, that's not what I want to do with my life."

"What *do* you want to do with your life?" I inquired gently.

He dropped his head just a little, almost apologetically, and color rushed to his cheeks. "I want to be a lawyer," he said, very, very quietly. "Like my dad."

And at that, his mother began to cry, too.

Jeff was facing a unique set of difficulties. On the one hand, he was virtually assured a college education. On the other hand, for him to reach his goal, he would have to actually perform in college. Football might get him through with a general liberal arts degree, but to be a lawyer he would have to go beyond that. He wouldn't be able to hide behind the misguided, albeit well-meaning, protection of his coaches or teachers. He would have to meet high academic expectations just to get into law school, then perform at an even more advanced level to succeed once he was accepted. He wouldn't be able to rely on his good looks and charming personality.

Jeff was aware of all of these things. Just as he was excruciatingly aware that his problems with reading and writing—his "hearing problem"—would pose substantial barriers to his ever being able to meet those expectations.

But at least now the disorder had a name. He could take comfort in the fact that he wasn't stupid as he had always feared. Instead, his difficulties had a very real physiologic cause. And we had agreed on an intensive plan of attack, including therapy techniques, environmental modification suggestions, and ways for him to compensate for his difficulties. When he left my office, he was once again smiling. This time it was a smile full of hope.

After intensive computer-based therapy, Jeff's reading decoding and auditory discrimination skills improved significantly. Acknowledging his disorder and giving it a name helped him to gain confidence in himself and his abilities. So, too, did teaching him to become an active listener and providing him with strategies to compensate for his disorder. Right now, Jeff is a sophomore in college, majoring in political science and playing football on a full-ride scholarship. He receives some special accommodations related to his disorder through the university's office of disabilities services, and he is earning solid A's and B's.

It wouldn't surprise me at all if Jeff did, indeed, finally make it to law school.

Jeff's story is somewhat typical of the children I see with APD. Many of them complain of difficulty with spelling and reading, inability to understand what is being said especially with noise in the background, and inner feelings of inadequacy and ignorance. Children with APD gradually become aware that something is wrong because they find themselves having to work so much harder at certain tasks than their friends do. Many children with APD, like Jeff, perform near enough to the normal range in school to disqualify them for special services. However, even those children who achieve some academic success usually come home from school at the end of every day exhausted from having to spend so much effort just listening. Then they are faced with several more grueling hours of effort to finish homework that might take their friends less than half that time to complete. Over time, they may learn to compensate to some degree for the disorder. But many children with APD continue to have problems into adulthood, especially if the disorder goes undiagnosed and untreated.

Also like Jeff, many children with APD become masters at hiding their disorder. In their early years, they may try to participate in conversations or classroom discussions; however, because their input is frequently off-topic or shows a lack of comprehension of the topic, they may be ridiculed, laughed at, or—even worse—simply ignored. After years of this, some children simply withdraw from communication altogether. Some become sullen and sit in their chairs with arms folded and hands fisted, belligerent scowls on their faces, daring anyone and everyone to attempt a connection. But this is merely a mask that allows them to protect their vulnerable, hidden inner selves and to retain some semblance of power over the daily situations in which they feel powerless. Although this frequently leads to social isolation, it is a self-imposed isolation and appears far more preferable and less humiliating to the child than the inevitable overt exclusion by others that they have experienced throughout their lives.

Others, like Jeff, continue to participate in life, to accumulate friends and join in extracurricular activities. This is particularly true for those children who exhibit some special talent in other areas such as sports, music, art, or theater. This special talent gives them an outlet for their need to connect with others while, at the same time, providing them with at least one environment in which they feel safe and can succeed. But even these children must deal with the frequent, and often unintentionally cruel, barbs from friends and teachers, the perception of them as somewhat "slow," the teasing that accompanies their frequent social and communicative faux pas—"Jeez, what are you, *stupid* or something?" So they, too, wear a mask of smiling tolerance and become the "good buddy" who'll put up with anything. And they frequently withdraw in their own way, becoming quiet followers in the parade of life, seemingly happy, sometimes even popular, but, all the while, bleeding inside.

CLAY: SEVERE APD IN A PRESCHOOLER

When he was really little, just a baby, Clay made all the same sounds that his sister made. We kept waiting for that first word to just pop out. But it never did. At first we thought, "Well, maybe it's because his sister is talking for him. I mean, she really does talk a lot." But he's four now. Four years old. And he doesn't understand us, and we don't understand him. Sometimes, when he's frustrated because he isn't getting what he wants, he just screams and screams and screams. At first they said he was autistic, then they said he was retarded. Now they just don't seem to know at all. We're starting to use sign language with him. What do you think? I'll learn sign language, I'll use it if that's what it takes. I just want to be able to talk with my baby. You know, sometimes I feel like screaming, too.

—Clay's mother

When I first saw Clay, he was four years old and had been in speech and language therapy for two years. His therapists and parents were working on basic skills such as teaching Clay to respond consistently to his name, repeat simple consonant-vowel syllables with visual cues, maintain appropriate eye contact, and follow simple commands. They were also augmenting his speech-language therapy with sign language, which he was beginning to pick up and use. The speech-language pathology supervisor, Sue, pulled me into the observation room one day to observe a therapy session. Except for his language development, everything about Clay argued that he was a normal little boy. He was curious, exhibited good motor skills, and played appropriately with toys. For example, when playing with a toy farm, he would place the farm animals where they belonged in their stalls or walk the little plastic cows around the pen outside the barn. He could put together puzzles, build things with blocks, and make toy airplanes "fly." He was affectionate and giggled when something amused him. Because of these behaviors, Clay's mother and Sue didn't think Clay was autistic or retarded. Beyond that, however, they had no idea what was causing Clay's speech and language delay. A developmental pediatrician had ruled out any medical or pathological cause for the delay, as well.

But Clay had virtually no receptive (understanding) or expressive (output) language. He was simply, in our terms, a "nonverbal child." He did not turn his head when his name was called. He did not follow even simple directions or answer questions like "How old are you?" or "What's your name?" He didn't name pictures in a book. He communicated only by gestures, grunts, and unrecognizable gibberish. He did not seem to have the basic understanding that speech has meaning and is important. As a result, he rarely even looked at the person who was talking to him.

When I observed Clay for the first time, I was struck by how similar his behavior was to that of a deaf child. He rarely responded to his name. He occasionally repeated portions of words or syllables, but he was neither consistent nor accurate with this skill. For example, if the speech-language pathologist said *pig* and pointed to a picture of a pig, Clay might respond with *ik, ig,* just the vowel itself, or nothing at all. On the other hand, when looking directly at the therapist and watching her mouth emphasize the *p* sound, complete with a dramatic release of air (which made him laugh), he would say "pig." But his spontaneous expressive communication consisted solely of grunts, points, and, as his mother described, screams when he was displeased.

Clay wasn't deaf. In fact, his hearing sensitivity was well within the normal range. He had been tested using what we call *conditioned play audiometry*—a test in which the child drops a block into a bucket in response to sound. By teaching Clay to drop a block whenever he heard beeps or tones of different pitches and loudness, we were able to determine the quietest sounds he could hear—or his hearing *thresholds*. We had obtained a complete audiogram, a graphic representation of Clay's thresholds from the low pitches all the way up to the high pitches. His hearing was entirely normal in both ears. Therefore, although he behaved precisely as we might expect a deaf child to behave, hearing loss was not the cause.

Yet, watching Clay that first time, I was convinced that, despite normal hearing sensitivity for tones, he *was,* for all intents and purposes, a deaf child.

Because of Clay's young age and lack of expressive abilities, we were unable to perform standard tests of auditory processing function with him. These tests require a mental age of seven or eight years, and the ability to repeat things such as numbers, words, and sentences. Diagnosis of APD is very difficult in children younger than about seven; however, there are other ways of determining how well a young child's auditory system and brain are able to cope with sound. One of these procedures uses *auditory electrophysiology.* For these tests, small electrodes are taped to various locations on the child's head, sounds are fed into the child's ears, and a computer screen records the brain's response to the sounds. The child must sit very still or be asleep for this testing. Unfortunately, deep sleep may abolish some of the responses from higher cortical regions of the brain that are dependent on consciousness. To get an active four-year-old to sit still while electrodes were applied to his scalp and sound was presented to his ears, I had Clay lie back in a chair with his mother and watch a favorite video. Because we were looking at brain-related responses to sound that don't require any conscious listening on the part of the child, the video did not interfere with the testing in any way. We obtained a clear picture of what we call the *neural representation* of sound from various portions of Clay's central auditory nervous system.

Results of Clay's testing indicated that the lower parts of his central auditory system, such as his brain stem, responded exactly as they should to sound. However, as we moved higher in the nervous system, the responses to sound began to diminish. Finally, at the level of the brain itself, or the cortical level, Clay's responses to sound were extremely reduced, especially over the left hemisphere of his brain, where actual speech-sound processing takes place.

All of this suggested that Clay exhibited a condition affecting basic neurophysiologic representation of sound at the cortical level of his brain. Although his young age may have affected these findings to a degree, that he was awake and alert during testing, combined with the presence of some response over the right side of his brain, was conclusive, physiologic evidence of an auditory processing deficit. In essence, although his ears were fine, his brain couldn't "hear" certain sounds.

"So he's deaf, after all?" his mother asked after the testing, some relief in her voice. This was not surprising because, as frightening as the presence of deafness in a child may be for a parent, at least such a clear-cut diagnosis would be understandable and would provide a definitive reason for Clay's speech delays. Even a diagnosis of deafness might be preferable to the endless lack of closure and understanding that results from never knowing why a child is having difficulties.

"No, not exactly," I explained. "He's not deaf in the traditional sense. In fact, his ears are functioning just fine. He hears sounds. He knows when the phone is ringing or someone is knocking at the door. He responds when the dog barks. He can hear your voice and it comforts and calms him. The problem is in the way his brain deals with sounds. It's probably hard for Clay's brain to interpret most of the sounds of speech. Even though he can hear someone talking to him, he can't really tell the difference—or discriminate—between the speech sounds themselves. He might hear everything muffled, like he's underwater. Or some speech sounds might sound just like others to him. He might not even truly understand that speech has meaning. It might all just be noise to him—like the dog barking or the knock on the door. That's why he doesn't understand what's said to him. It's also why he doesn't speak clearly, because our ability to speak is closely tied to our ability to hear."

"It's because he had so many ear infections when he was a baby, isn't it?" Clay's mother asked. "The doctor told me they wouldn't affect his development, but I was always worried about them."

I explained that, although a link has been shown between a history of early, chronic ear infections and auditory processing problems in some children, there was no way of knowing how much these infections had contributed to Clay's difficulties. Certainly, if ear infections occur frequently enough at a very young age, the child often misses some of the speech and language input during those periods that are critical for language development. On the other hand, many children have a history of severe ear infections throughout their childhood and exhibit no lasting effects whatsoever. Furthermore, for many children, ear infections may be "silent"—that is, without evidence of pain or fever—and thus go undetected for a long time. In these children, it is difficult to determine in hindsight to what degree the infections may have affected the child's language and learning.

We simply do not know why the vast majority of APD cases occur. That is one of the hardest things for a parent of a child with an APD to accept: the realization that the underlying cause, the why of it all, will likely never be identified. We do know, however, that many cases of APD are present very early in life, probably at birth. They don't just develop suddenly, unless the child has had some type of head injury, illness, or other trauma that can affect brain function.

Over the summer, Clay underwent intensive auditory training, both computer-based and interactive, focusing in tandem on both discriminating (telling the difference between) and producing (speaking) speech sounds. Most of these games required Clay to imitate consonants, vowels, syllables, and words presented by animated characters on a computer screen. When he responded correctly, the characters rewarded him with music and dancing. By the end of the summer, his ability to imitate syllables, words, and even short phrases had improved remarkably. His spontaneous expressive vocabulary began to increase as well. When he returned to the clinic in the fall after a short hiatus, he surprised all of us by greeting me in the hallway with the words, "Hi, teacher."

When I wrote the first draft of this chapter, Clay's story stopped here. I knew that Clay's student clinicians would continue to work with him on speech and language production as well as auditory skills during the fall semester. I knew that some progress would be seen, but I couldn't predict just how far he would go or whether he would ever exhibit normal speech and language skills. However, those two words—"Hi, teacher"—had given us all reason to hope.

Near the end of the fall semester, Sue once again pulled me into the observation room to watch a therapy session. On the other side of the one-way glass, I saw Clay and his clinician playing a game that used blocks and action cards to help put words in their correct order in sentences. I watched as Clay spontaneously produced four-word sentences, imitated eight-word sentences, and laughed and chattered with the clinician, clearly enjoying his newly acquired ability to communicate.

Just a few short months ago this child had been virtually nonverbal. Now, for the first time, Clay was able to communicate his true nature. Witty, affectionate, funny, and bright, his delightful personality shone through in his words and actions. It was as if he had finally become aware that sound had meaning, and because of that awareness, the floodgates had opened, allowing language to flow through him. We stood in the darkness—Sue and I—watching this miracle and cried.

And we thought, "This is what it's all about. This is why we do what we do. One child like this—just one—makes everything we do worthwhile."

A few weeks later, I reevaluated Clay's brain responses to sound. They looked entirely normal for a four-year-old child. He still needed therapy to improve his pronunciation—or articulation—of speech sounds and to build his language skills. But his accomplishments in a very short period of time were nothing short of remarkable.

LARRY: MILD APD IN AN ADULT

Not all people with auditory processing deficits exhibit obvious and severe difficulties during early childhood. In some cases, APD does not manifest itself until much later in life and, even then, sometimes not until the conditions are precisely right:

I never had any problems in school. Not that I was a star student or anything, but I got by just fine. Got my MBA, but after a few years in the corporate world, I got bored. Guess I needed more action. I'd done some investing over the years, mostly on-line, and I thought the whole stock market thing was fascinating. So I went for it. During our training, we were allowed to go down onto the trade floor—what an exciting place! I couldn't really understand a lot of what was going on, but I figured that I just had a lot to learn. When it came my turn to take my spot on that floor, I was really nervous. People were waving papers and yelling things at me. I couldn't understand anything. My boss told me that it wasn't unusual for someone to freak out the first time or two they're in the action like that. But the problem wouldn't go away. I've got all the skills, I know what to look for, I know how and when to trade, damn it! But, down there, when they're all yelling at me like that and I'm supposed to react fast, I just can't do it. I can't seem to make sense of all the noise and the chaos. They pulled me off the floor and I'm at a desk job now. They're even talking about firing me. I've never been fired in my life! I really thought I'd like this field, really looked forward to being where all the action is. But how will I ever know if I can't even do it, if I'm stuck behind a desk? I might as well go back to corporate management.

—Larry

Larry was referred to me by his employer after another audiologist had determined that his actual hearing acuity was normal and suggested the possibility of an APD. By the time I saw him, he was frustrated and somewhat defensive because of the treatment he had been receiving lately from his supervisor. Although his boss had been understanding at first, Larry was now becoming a liability to the company and was on the verge of being fired. He was forty-three years old and was looking at being unemployed with a wife, two children, and a house in the burbs. It was a potentially volcanic situation.

Larry's testing revealed a very mild auditory processing deficit specifically in his ability to "fill in" missing pieces of a message—a process we refer to as *auditory closure.* He also had difficulty with messages in general when they were presented in competing conditions, such as when different information was given to each ear at the same time. It was unclear whether Larry had had this mild disorder all of his life or if it was adult-onset. What was clear was that his deficit was so mild that it would have been no more than an occasional, mild annoyance in typical situations. The only environments in which Larry would have noticed his mild deficit would have been those where the background noise level was extremely high—such as on the floor of the stock exchange.

Larry's case illustrates that even a very mild auditory deficit can nevertheless be extremely disruptive depending on the unique circumstances of a person's life. Larry would have been successful in virtually any other job, as he had proven prior to his career change. However, when he paired his auditory deficit with the unusual and extreme auditory demands of working on a trade floor, he was unable to perform. Larry couldn't have made a worse career choice given his particular auditory disorder.

Larry was forced to accept that he could never compensate sufficiently for his mild deficit to be able to perform in an environment like the stock exchange. He has moved back to the corporate business world and, last I heard, was doing quite well. But I am sure he still thinks occasionally about the color and excitement of the world he left behind.

Larry's situation brings to light one unfortunate but very real factor that must be considered in any discussion of APD. Although treatment may remediate the disorder, some residual difficulty may well continue for the remainder of the person's life. When we develop a management program for APD, we address these issues and suggest methods of compensating for the residual disorder as well as strategies for changing the listening environment to make it more friendly for the person with APD. However, even with such strategies in place, the individual may simply have to accept that he will have difficulty in some situations. This was precisely the case with Larry and the stock exchange. The very nature of his job setting made any environmental changes impossible and rendered his compensatory strategies virtually ineffective. He was forced to make a realistic life choice—to change his job setting entirely.

Individuals with APD must realize that, just as with other disabilities, some activities will continue to be difficult or impossible, depending on the severity of the disorder. Although we do not wish to dampen anyone's dreams or to encourage individuals with APD to limit themselves unnecessarily, we must also be practical. When one considers the frustration and self-flagellation that is almost unavoidable when one sets unattainable goals and continually, without exception, fails, then perhaps it is time to choose a different objective, one that is no less enticing but is more likely to be within reach.

JASON: RIGHT-HEMISPHERE DISORDER AND APD

All three of the cases presented thus far have focused on the effects of auditory processing disorder on the perception of speech sounds. The dysfunction could be localized, generally, to the language-dominant (or left) hemisphere of the brain, where speech-sound analysis and representation takes place. However, not all auditory processing disorders arise from left-hemisphere dysfunction. Nor do all auditory processing disorders affect the perception of speech per se. The auditory manifestations of dysfunction in the right side of the brain can frequently be just as pervasive, and harder to pin down, as those of left-hemisphere dysfunction. Furthermore, in many cases, right-hemisphere dysfunction can lead to other disorders and difficulties that have a devastating impact on the individual's social, communicative, and psychological well-being:

Jason doesn't have any friends. I mean that. No friends at all. No one likes him. He doesn't do anything that I see other little boys do. He doesn't like puzzles, never played with LEGOs or blocks. Half the time, he just sits there. It's like he's drugged or something. We try to joke with him, but he just looks at us with that stony face—like a robot. Sometimes he'll laugh a little, like when he's watching a Three Stooges movie or something. I love it when he laughs. But most of the time he just seems so depressed. He does all right in school, and all of the testing says that his learning abilities are normal, that there's nothing wrong with him. So they won't even do anything. They just said that he has emotional problems, like his brothers, and leave it at that. Maybe it's us, maybe we've done something wrong. You know, his older brother is in a special home for kids with emotional problems. And his oldest brother, well, you probably already know about him from the report. I don't know. I just don't think I can take this anymore. What are we doing wrong?

—Jason's mother

Jason was a handsome little eight-year-old boy. He lived in a small state where no auditory processing services were available, and I was brought out to assess several children suspected of auditory deficit. Jason was a last-minute addition to my assessment list. His referral to me resulted less from any obvious auditory difficulty than from desperation on the part of the private psychologist working with him to uncover any information at all that might help explain this enigmatic child. Unlike with most of the children I assess, I hadn't had much opportunity to review Jason's records, and frankly, I was a little unsure as to the appropriateness of the referral. Despite my misgivings, I agreed to test him.

The little information I had been able to glean from his records indicated no obvious learning or language difficulties. The speech-language report did say, however, that he exhibited mild pragmatic concerns—or concerns regarding his *use* of language, particularly relating to social communication. Jason didn't seem to understand quite what to do or say in a social situation. He might interrupt or show other signs of inappropriate turn-taking behaviors. Although his contributions to a conversation were generally related to the topic of discussion, he would stray from the key point and end up talking about something that really wasn't the focus of the conversation. For example, during a conversation about endangered species, Jason might begin talking about the bald eagle, but somehow work his way around to a discussion of his pet cat. He often failed to laugh at jokes, overreacted to perceived insults or sarcasm, and ignored social conventions such as making expected responses to salutations ("Hello, how are you?" "I'm fine, thank you. How are you?") or saying good-bye appropriately ("It was good to see you. Have a nice day").

Furthermore, his speech-language pathologist stated that Jason's expressive speech was not abnormal exactly, but was a little, well, *unusual*. She couldn't quite put her finger on it, but his rhythm and cadence were subtly wrong somehow. Just a little off in some indefinable way. He didn't speak in a monotone exactly, but he didn't seem as animated as most boys his age. More obvious was his lack of facial expression. This latter finding was also characteristic of depression, something that was prevalent in Jason's family. Both of his older brothers had been diagnosed with depressive disorders. The middle boy had attempted suicide when he was ten years old and was currently living in a group home for children with emotional disturbances. The oldest boy, tragically, had killed himself at the age of fourteen.

Jason was under the care of a psychologist when I saw him, but he wasn't receiving any special services in school because he didn't exhibit any documented language or learning deficits that would qualify him for special education in those areas. He wasn't great at math, but fell loosely within the low end of the normal range. His nonverbal IQ scores were lower than his verbal scores, but not significantly so. He was, however, classified as emotionally disturbed and received some accommodations in the classroom due to that.

During testing, Jason offered none of the chitchat that typically accompanies my evaluations with children, even though he understood all of the directions easily and was entirely compliant. On some of the testing, Jason performed just fine, well within the normal range for his age. Yet he had a good deal of difficulty with certain tasks when competing messages were delivered to both ears at the same time. More revealing, he could not perform at all during a task that required him not to repeat speech sounds, but to perceive subtle pitch and duration differences in sequences of tones or beeps. This required the right side of his brain to hear the pattern, or acoustic contour, of the tones. Jason understood the task, could describe the patterns easily when the differences between stimuli were large or when I "sang" them in my own voice. But when the differences were subtle, he reported that the tones all sounded the same.

This pattern of performance indicated an auditory processing disorder, but Jason's specific type of APD was not in discriminating speech sounds or other "left-brain" auditory skills. Rather, his difficulty, like my own, was in those "right-brain" auditory abilities that are responsible for perceiving nonspeech or "musical" aspects of the signal, including those cues that convey tone of voice and assist us in understanding what is *meant* in relation to what is *said.* People with this type of auditory disorder frequently misunderstand the intent of others' communications, often complain of hurt feelings, and may themselves speak in a monotone or with little expression. Often, the cadence or rhythm of their expressive speech is somewhat distorted, as was Jason's. This type of deficit may affect a person's ability to appreciate humor or sarcasm, to engage in socially appropriate conversational exchanges with others, and to "read between the lines." These abilities come naturally to most, and they help to make communication the many-layered, enjoyable activity it usually is. But for a child or adult with right-hemisphere-based APD, communication is far from enjoyable. It can be a painful, frequently embarrassing, or confusing experience.

And yet, Jason's auditory processing deficits were, without question, the least of his concerns. My testing had uncovered merely the auditory piece of what was clearly a more global right-hemisphere deficit that affected Jason's functioning in many other areas. Jason's symptoms made me suspect a disorder that is sometimes referred to as *nonverbal learning disability* or NVLD. NVLD can lead to a wide variety of symptoms including social difficulties, depression, difficulty with nonverbal tasks (including math calculation and visual-spatial activities), expressive and receptive prosody (or tone of voice) difficulties, allocation of attention, and the like. All of these symptoms appeared to be present to some degree in Jason's case. Certainly, however, his depression was of primary and immediate concern, particularly given his family history. It is possible that Jason's depression was exacerbated by his lack of success in socialization and communication. But because depression frequently co-occurs with right-hemisphere dysfunction, it is difficult to determine just how much of Jason's emotional difficulties were linked to his auditory processing deficit.

I referred Jason to a university center where cutting-edge research into NVLD was being undertaken. They confirmed other, more subtle diagnostic indicators of right-hemisphere dysfunction, such as that Jason exhibited a lesser degree of visual scanning to the left of center as compared to the right of center as measured by infrared tracking of his eye movements. Auditory and related testing eventually completed on Jason's older brother revealed the same pattern.

Jason is currently undergoing therapy for both visual-spatial abilities and auditory perception and production of prosodic aspects of speech. He and his brother are being closely monitored by a team of psychiatrists, and trials with antidepressant medication have been initiated. When he entered the fourth grade and the learning demands increased, Jason began to exhibit clear difficulties in mathematics, so he is now receiving special services for these and related academic difficulties.

I don't know that it's accurate to state that Jason exhibits a primary auditory processing disorder. Certainly, his performance yielded clear patterns consistent with an APD; however, this was just one small factor contributing to Jason's overall difficulties. Of far more concern were the emotional and psychological manifestations of Jason's, and his brother's, right-hemisphere involvement. Importantly, the results of central auditory testing provided information that allowed us to explore further, and ultimately uncover, the underlying problem.

I also don't know to what extent therapy will be effective for Jason's difficulties. Most of the research into auditory and related therapy efficacy has focused on speech-sound training and left-hemisphere disorders. I hope that he can learn ways in which to compensate for his difficulties. I also hope that psychiatric and pharmacological interventions will address his emotional and depressive disorders sufficiently. But Jason may always have some difficulty judging communicative intent and comprehending the subtle, prosody-related, and social aspects of communication.

Jason's situation emphasizes some important principles of APD that should be understood. First, not all auditory processing disorders are speech-sound related. A person may be able to tell the difference between speech sounds well, be able to spell and write fluently, yet still exhibit auditory processing problems. More important, even if a child exhibits a clear auditory processing deficit, that deficit may not be the only, or even the most important, factor contributing to his or her learning or communication problems.

Many disorders either mimic APD or can coexist with APD, such as attention-deficit/hyperactivity disorder (AD/HD), autism, NVLD, and similar conditions. Confirming the presence of an APD in these cases is important; however, the diagnosis of an APD as a coexisting condition should not be taken to mean that all of the individual's difficulties can, therefore, be attributed to the auditory disorder. Instead, it is more often the case that the auditory disorder is merely one piece of the overall picture. As in Jason's case, APD may not even be the most important piece when one considers the individual as a whole. We must consider auditory processing in the context of larger, more global disorders that can affect a person's daily life skills and coping strategies in a variety of ways.

Furthermore, as Jason's case illustrates, APD diagnostic services may not be available in a given geographic locale. In recent years, the increased attention and education devoted to APD has resulted in increased APD services throughout this country and abroad. However, not all audiologists are educated or trained in diagnosis or management of APD, nor should they be expected to be. APD requires a specialized degree of expertise that goes beyond that provided in our typical audiological training programs.

EVELYN: APD IN THE ELDERLY

If it hasn't already been apparent, it should be pointed out that all of the preceding stories have dealt with males. Auditory processing disorders like learning disabilities, occur in males more frequently than in females, but they can and do occur in females. Furthermore, although the cases discussed so far have exhibited normal hearing sensitivity, auditory processing disorders can coexist with hearing loss, which can make management of the hearing loss more difficult:

> *Don't like them. Take them away. I can't hear any better with the dang things than I can without them. Everything's just noise. Noise, noise, noise. Gives me a headache trying to make sense of all that noise.*
>
> —*Evelyn*

Evelyn was a small, white-haired, seventy-four-year-old woman who had absolutely no compunctions about expressing her true feelings. She had a pretty typical age-related hearing impairment that led to difficulties understanding speech, especially in noise or at church. She had recently been fitted with hearing aids in both ears after finally being convinced by her daughter-in-law to do something about her progressive hearing loss.

But the hearing aids didn't seem to help Evelyn. Nothing did. Whether she wore her hearing aids or not, Evelyn complained that she still couldn't understand what people were saying. The problem, she insisted, wasn't hearing, it was understanding. The hearing aids just made everything louder, not clearer.

Evelyn was referred to me because the standard hearing testing done before she was fit with hearing aids didn't explain why she was having such significant difficulties. In fact, her ability to hear and understand words was quite good when she was tested one ear at a time using headphones. This suggested that Evelyn would be an excellent candidate for binaural amplification—hearing aids in both ears. Although some tests of auditory processing require that the listener's hearing be normal, some do not. I administered those central auditory tests that were appropriate for people with hearing impairment to get an idea of what other factors, not related to Evelyn's hearing loss, might be contributing to her listening difficulties.

Evelyn had far greater difficulty than other women her age during tasks in which competing messages were delivered to both ears at the same time. She also had difficulty with the tonal patterns tests described in the previous case, but unlike Jason, she could hear the differences among the stimuli just fine and was able to hum them with the conviction of a church choir leader, which, incidentally, she was. She could not, however, label or verbally describe them (e.g., high-high-low or long-short-long) when asked to do so. Memory was not an issue here. Evelyn was, and still is, sharp as a tack and can repeat entire strings of numbers or words on demand, as long as the numbers or words are presented in noncompeting conditions. No, Evelyn's difficulties stemmed from the fact that these dichotic listening and tonal patterns tests relied on the ability of both hemispheres of the brain to communicate with one another.

Recent research into auditory processing and aging has indicated that the ability of the two hemispheres of the brain to cooperate—interhemispheric integration—decreases significantly as we age. Furthermore, the data suggest that this integration deficit, if sufficiently pronounced, may well affect our binaural listening abilities, including the benefit we receive from binaural hearing aids. Evelyn's pattern of findings on central auditory testing confirmed that she exhibited just such a pronounced integration deficit. As she had insisted, the problem really wasn't her hearing. It was her ability to understand—especially when both ears (and therefore, both hemispheres of her brain) were being forced to work together.

Although most people do hear better with two hearing aids—a situation that most closely resembles normal hearing—we discovered that Evelyn heard much better when she wore only one hearing aid in her right ear. She returned the left hearing aid and marched away happily, right hearing aid in place and turned up good and high. It's a Sunday morning as I write this, and I'm certain that at this very moment Evelyn is singing happily in the church choir or listening to the minister's sermon, quite satisfied with herself that she hadn't paid for two hearing aids when she does just fine, even better, with one.

Evelyn exhibited a third type of auditory processing problem, one in which the issue is neither "left-brain" nor "right-brain," but rather the way in which the two hemispheres of the brain interact. This common type of APD occurs in children as well as adults. In Evelyn's case, most of her difficulty was auditory in nature. However, many people with this type of integration deficit have difficulty with virtually any task that requires cooperation between the two halves of the brain and may exhibit what are commonly called sensory integration issues. From an auditory perspective, not only may they have difficulty with understanding speech in noise and telling where a sound is coming from, but they may have difficulty in linking the "left-brain" speech sound and language functions with the "right-brain" tone-of-voice or prosodic cues, resulting in some confusion and miscomprehension of what is being said *and* meant. The auditory manifestations of integration deficit may be extremely disruptive, or they may be relatively mild when compared to the sensory integration symptoms. Therefore, once again, we must consider the whole person to determine the degree to which a given APD may be affecting someone's life, for it is this picture that should guide our treatment efforts.

IF A TREE FALLS IN THE FOREST: DEBATING THE EXISTENCE OF APD

It is not always possible to demonstrate objectively the presence of an APD. In fact, in many cases of APD, physiologic tests such as brain scans, electrophysiology, and magnetic resonance imaging (MRI) fail to reveal any obvious structural or functional damage or dysfunction. This not only poses a difficulty for audiologists in diagnosing APD (particularly in the case of very young children who cannot yet participate in behavioral testing), but also leads to denial on the part of some medical and other professionals that APD exists at all. Tragically, the assertion "If you can't see it, it isn't there" has led some to conclude that APD, very simply, is not real.

If a tree falls in the forest and no one is around to hear it fall, does it make a sound? Although people love to debate the two possible answers to this question, it is not really a philosophical question at all. And there is only one correct answer.

The definition of sound is "a propogation of vibration through a sound-conducting medium." Therefore, unless the tree is in outer space or in a vacuum, in which there is no sound-conducting medium such as air, of course it makes a sound. That no one is around to hear it fall is completely irrelevant and, thus, should not even enter into the equation.

Case closed. End of discussion.

Still, some continue to debate this issue, just as some contend that, if no one is around to understand, test for, or treat auditory processing disorders, or if they do not show up on our brain scans or other physiologic tests, then they, likewise, do not exist.

On the face of it, this argument seems reasonable, logical even. Logical, that is, until we consider the limitations of current medical procedures and technology in detecting subtle abnormalities in function as well as structure of anatomical organs. The brain is highly complex, with infinitesimal biomolecular and neurochemical influences that shape the function of the nervous system. It is not at all surprising that physical evidence of specific damage or dysfunction is lacking for the majority of APD cases. Indeed, it would be more surprising if all of these difficulties had a clearly evident, easily defined underlying cause.

For years, professionals and scientists have looked for the specific physiologic causes responsible for such conditions as autism, schizophrenia, learning disabilities, mental retardation, language delays, dyslexia, attention -deficit/hyperactivity disorder, and many other disabilities. And for years, those visible, documentable signs have eluded all of us. But we continue to search. We don't simply refuse to acknowledge their existence.

Not so with auditory processing disorders. From the first proposal of the term APD to describe these hearing deficits in the 1960s, the existence argument has raged. Some have said that auditory processing deficits are merely a manifestation of a specific learning disability or attention deficit or language disorder. Some have said that the frequent coexistence, or *comorbidity*, of auditory deficits with these other disorders render them merely one characteristic of a larger, more global disability. Some have even said that there is no way in which an auditory-based deficit of any type can have the kind of far-reaching implications hypothesized by the pro-APD camp.

Many of these arguments have arisen, no doubt, from at least some degree of professional territorialism and defensiveness. After all, many professionals in the field of speech, language, and learning had been working with these difficulties long before they ever had a formal label. Why, now, after all these years, should we suddenly "invent" a new label for an old set of problems that may well just be manifestations of other disorders already understood and diagnosable?

When confronted with the existence argument from fellow professionals, I offer the following response derived from current research into APD:

- Some children and adults exhibit extreme difficulties in primarily, if not solely, the auditory modality that affect their day-to-day communication and learning abilities.

- For the majority of these individuals, hearing loss simply cannot account for their difficulties.

- These individuals exhibit specific patterns of findings on tests of central auditory function that precisely mirror those of known pathologies involving the central auditory nervous system *and nothing else,* which cannot be ignored or put down merely to coincidence.

- A growing body of evidence obtained from new technological measures of auditory processing is demonstrating that the neural representation of sound in the higher brain stem or brain pathways of many of these individuals simply is different from that of other, nondisordered individuals.

In short, the battle over the existence of auditory processing deficits has begun to abate under the pressure of such overwhelming evidence. Although it is still possible to encounter someone in the fields of medicine or psychology or education or speech-language pathology or even audiology who asserts, "APD doesn't exist, and even if it did, there's nothing we can do about it anyway," this statement is, thankfully, far less frequent today than even just five short years ago.

As more information becomes available, as more sharing of findings and ideas is fostered among professionals in many different disciplines, and as new technological advances continue to support the existence of auditory deficits that can, indeed, impact a wide variety of functional areas, it is my fondest hope that this futile debate will end.

In the meantime, if a tree falls in the forest and no one is around to hear it fall, does it make a sound? You bet.

You've met several people each of whom exhibited an auditory processing disorder that affected his or her life in vastly different ways. I hope that their stories have convinced you that not only are auditory processing disorders very real, but that they may occur in anyone, at any age, and may manifest themselves in various manners. The stories you have read do not even come close to representing all of the possible combinations of gender, age, central auditory findings, and impact on life skills that are possible. They serve merely to illustrate the heterogeneous, complex nature of the disorder.

In the early days of APD, a definition of auditory processing was proposed by Dr. Jack Katz of Buffalo, New York. He stated that auditory processing could be defined as "what we do with what we hear." Over time, we have tried to hone this definition, to render it scientifically more technical, to narrow it down to specific auditory mechanisms. Also, because of the difficulty in developing a precise definition of what APD is and what it isn't, we have argued endlessly over what to call it, and by the time this book goes to press, our label for this disorder may have changed yet again. But, despite our best efforts, the heterogeneous and interactive nature of auditory processing deficits has eluded our grasp so that no specific definition of or label for auditory processing and its disorders has successfully captured its true essence. Therefore, we now are witnessing a re-evolution in which we are acknowledging that auditory processing does, indeed, consist of "what we do with what we hear." In a sense, we have come full circle, but now we are armed with more ammunition with which to analyze and fight the beast.

However, despite our increased knowledge, our ever-improving tools and measures and tests, we still have much to learn. In truth, what we do not know about auditory processing far outweighs what is in our current realm of understanding. In this fascinating, frustrating, and complex area, we still have, in the timeless words of Robert Frost, "miles to go before we sleep."

LEARNING, LANGUAGE, AND AUDITORY PROCESSING

No two people will react to the presence of an APD in precisely the same way. For some people, APD is clearly a disorder of *hearing*. That is, the person is aware that he has difficulty hearing or listening that is worse in some situations than in others, and that interferes with the ability to understand what is said. For others, however, the actual hearing—or listening—difficulties that arise from APD are much more subtle and far less disruptive than the effects those same auditory difficulties have on other life skills, such as learning, language, spelling, reading, socializing, and problem-solving. In this chapter, we will discuss the relationship between APD and these other, seemingly unrelated, areas.

First, however, several considerations, or principles, should be kept in mind. These principles are based on the science and theory of what APD is and how it relates to various other functions in the brain. By understanding these principles and keeping them in mind at all times, we will avoid the tendency to attribute any and all disorders involving learning, language, and related abilities to APD.

Principle number one: *When we say auditory processing disorder, we really do mean AUDITORY.* In other words, when we discuss APD, we are referring to a problem or dysfunction in the auditory system—specifically, the *central* auditory system, or the portion of the system that runs from the ear to the brain. We are not referring to ear-based auditory problems, such as hearing loss or deafness, although hearing loss will certainly have an impact on the ability to listen, learn, and process language. We are also not referring to higher-level thinking or attention problems, such as mental retardation, autism, or AD/HD, even though these disorders, too, will affect listening and related skills and may even co-exist with or mimic APD. When we refer to APD, we are referring to primarily an "input" disorder that affects specifically the way auditory information is processed at a variety of levels in the central auditory nervous system.

Principle number two: Hearing, thinking, and attention abilities are still important. Disorders of the ear or higher-level cognitive or attention deficits are not to be confused with APD. Nevertheless, we must acknowledge that these disorders, when they coexist with APD, will add significantly, even multiplicatively, to the learning, language, and communication difficulties the person will have. For example, the presence of excellent higher-order memory, thinking, and attention skills provides a person with considerable strengths upon which to draw to compensate for lower-level auditory processing difficulties. On the other hand, if a deficit also exists in these higher-order abilities, the person's ability to rely on these skills will be lessened, rendering the auditory deficit more destructive. Similarly, a hearing loss in someone with an APD will result in greater difficulty in listening and comprehending than would the presence of an APD alone.

Principle number three: Not every language or learning problem is an APD. When we consider the relationship between APD and language or learning problems, we must realize that the issues are complex, involving the entire system, from the ear to the highest possible levels of thought and attention in the brain. We are also dealing with the integration of information from many different sensory systems. It must be emphasized that, while APD may affect a child's ability to learn to read or spell, *not all spelling or reading disorders are due to APD.* Similarly, although APD in a child will often have a devastating effect on language and speaking abilities, *not all receptive or expressive language disorders are due to APD.* Finally, although APD may affect problem-solving and socialization abilities, *difficulties in these areas may be due to many factors other than APD.*

A IS FOR *APPLE:* AUDITORY PROCESSING AND SPELLING

Think back to how you learned to spell. No doubt one technique you used was to associate speech sounds with the letters of the alphabet. For example, to read the word *dog,* you said the *d* sound, the *o* sound, and the *g* sound, then put it all together: D . . . O . . . G, DOG! This "sounding-out," or *phonics,* approach, is a standard method used to teach children how to spell and has been featured in many popular spelling and reading programs.

Imagine, now, that you do not hear the speech sounds correctly. For example, you find it difficult to discriminate between a *d* or a *g*—they sound the same to you. Therefore, the word *dog* might sound like *gog, God,* or *dod.* It would then become difficult to determine which letters of the alphabet you should choose to spell a given word—an alphabet that consists of twenty-six symbols, each of which must be recognized and memorized. Moreover, some speech sounds in the English language can be represented by several different letters, depending on the situation. The *s* sound, for example, can be represented by *s* in *bus,* by *ss* in *kiss,* by *c* in *city,* and so on. Similarly, the *j* sound is represented by both *j* and *dg,* sometimes even in the same word, such as *judge.* Sometimes it seems surprising that a child can learn to spell at all. Thus, although spelling appears simple, it is a complex task involving hearing, vision, and higher-level processing, memory, and integration abilities.

The phonics approach to spelling relies on some important assumptions. Foremost is the assumption that the child can both hear and discriminate among the various speech sounds that occur in our language. This is a prerequisite for success in this type of spelling, for sounding out words is based almost entirely on this skill. Second, the phonics approach assumes that the child has the necessary visual perceptual skills to recognize and discriminate between the patterns of lines and curves on a page—the orthographic symbols—that make up the individual letters of the alphabet. Finally, the phonics approach assumes that the child will be able to learn and remember how to associate the sound she hears with the symbol on the page, which requires integration of auditory and visual inputs. This process is called *sound-symbol association*. Spelling difficulties can arise from difficulties with the sound, the symbol, or with the association between the two. Deficits in any of these areas will result in difficulty learning to spell.

That spelling relies heavily on how we hear the speech sounds is demonstrated by the frequent use of "invented spelling" in today's elementary-school classrooms. Any parent with a young child in an early-elementary school grade probably has a paper similar to the following tacked up on the refrigerator door:

> *My favrit pursun in the wurd is my mom. She koks for me and I luv the peesa with peprone on it. I luv my dog. But I dont lik it win my dog ets my peesa. I luv my bruter to but he ets my peesa and I hit him. I haf to go to tim owt win I hit my bruter. I dont lik tim owt. My dad is my favrit pursn to. He lets me owt of tim owt win mom is mad. He plaz basbal wit me.*

This is an excellent example of emerging phonics-based spelling skills in a young school-aged child. Although many of the words are technically misspelled, the entire communication can be read and understood quite easily. Most of the words are spelled exactly as they sound, something that probably makes more sense than the irregular and confusing spelling rules that exist in the English language.

"Invented spelling" samples such as these can provide extraordinary insight into how the child hears the sounds of speech. Unlike the child whose writing is featured above, a child with a speech-sound-based

APD would have difficulty with this type of writing. Furthermore, understanding this child's invented spelling would likely be much more difficult. A child's inability to perform invented spelling at a young age may be an early "red flag" of an APD.

Remember, however, that spelling does not rely on speech-sound processing alone. The child must also remember the symbol or symbols that represent each speech sound and associate the two. Finally, spelling is essentially an "output" behavior requiring the child to *do* something to demonstrate his or her skills. That is, the child must integrate all of this knowledge and, using both memory and planning, write the letters in the correct order on a page or say them out loud. Just as deficits in the sounds, the symbols, or the association may interfere with the child's ability to grasp the underlying premise of spelling, deficits in memory or planning (two abilities that fall under the general cognitive umbrella of *executive function*) will also interfere with the ability to articulate, either on paper or aloud, what the child has internalized. And this is all assuming that the child has sufficient allocation of attention (another executive function) to devote to complete the task!

In trying to unravel this issue, I frequently look at writing samples of children and analyze their spelling errors for evidence of possible acoustic confusions rather than other types of difficulties. Acoustic confusions arise from sounds that are so close together that a child with speech-sound APD would likely hear them interchangeably or not be able to discriminate between them at all. Classic examples of these are consonants such as *b, d, g, p, t,* and *k.*

These consonants are so similar because of the patterns of sound that they make. The difference between a *d* and a *g,* for example, consists only of a very minute difference in the frequency (spectral) and timing (temporal) characteristics of the sound. Think of a continuum, with the syllable *da* at one end and *ga* at the other. If we begin to alter the precise frequency and timing of these sounds, using synthesized speech and a specialized computer program, the *da* will begin to sound less *da*-like and the *ga* will begin to sound less *ga*-like. Ultimately, the two will meet in the middle of the continuum and there will be no difference between them. They will sound the same.

People who process sounds normally are able to tell the difference between *d* and *g* even when they are pretty close together on that continuum. Recent research by Dr. Nina Kraus and her colleagues at the Northwestern University Auditory Neuroscience Laboratory has shown, however, that for some children with learning, language, and reading/spelling difficulties, these sounds must be much farther apart on the continuum to be distinguished. Indeed, research at Kraus's laboratory on recordings of brain-wave activity that relates to speech-sound discrimination has shown that the brains of these children do not show the pattern of discrimination found in normal listeners.

On the other hand, the difference between *b* and *w* is larger and relates to the length (or duration) of spectral changes in the speech sounds. This is a much easier discrimination to make and, indeed, appears to occur at a more basic, lower level than the cortex of the brain. The Northwestern studies show that children who have difficulty discriminating *d* and *g* have no difficulty with *b* and *w*. This finding is accompanied by the expected, normal brain-wave discrimination response for *b/w* in these children.

What does all of this mean for the real world? When each consonant is at its own far end of the continuum, we would consider that an exemplar—or perfect example—of the speech sound. In daily speech, we rarely talk using exemplars. Our words may be slurred or mumbled or the speech sounds may be altered slightly because of what sounds have occurred before or will occur after each one. In other words, these speech sounds in daily conversation usually fall somewhere toward the middle of the continuum rather than at the ends. For a child with normal processing abilities, this does not pose much of a problem. A *d* still sounds like a *d* and a *g* still sounds like a *g* even when they are rather close on the continuum. For the child with speech-sound-based APD, however, those sounds may seem the same much of the time. And, if they sound the same, they may be used interchangeably when the child is spelling. The child may even substitute one for the other in speaking. These speech-sound confusions will certainly have an effect on how well the child or adult is able to comprehend what is being said.

When I look for auditory confusions in invented or regular spelling samples, I am searching for errors that would be logical if the child is having difficulty discriminating among speech sounds, or hearing speech as somewhat "slurred" or unclear. I would expect the letters to be in approximately the correct order (e.g., consonant, vowel, consonant), but certain letters might be substituted for others that sound similar, and some may be deleted. Other words might be run together, as frequently happens in speech. The sample might still be readable but will not be as "logical" from an auditory perspective.

Consider the following example. The text is the same as in the child's passage previously presented, but taken from a spelling sample of a second-grade girl with a left-hemisphere, speech-sound-based APD:

> *My vavd besn ina wud is my mum. She kig fr me anl luv the bese wit brone ont. I luv my dug. But I don lit itin my dug et my pese. I luv my bute to bu het my pese anl item. I af tigo tenod hin I et my bute. I dunlit tenod. My dad is my vaved besn to. e lid me od tenod in mom is med. e pa bebal wime.*

The letters follow a logical consonant-vowel-consonant progression, for the most part. However, many letters are substituted with inaccurate ones, and clear demarcation between many of the words is missing. If we were to read this sample aloud, it might sound somewhat like slurred or distorted speech . . . which, in this case, is precisely how our testing indicated that this child was hearing speech in her daily life.

In contrast to the above sample, children with more visual-based spelling disorders may actually use the correct letters, but either write them backward or transpose the order of the letters in the word. Writing letters backward (for example, *b/d*) is quite common when children are just learning to write, but is much more pervasive and frequent when a child has a visual processing problem that affects the way he or she actually sees the symbols and words on the page. In addition, if the child has difficulty in output planning, the letters on the page may merely be jumbled, with no rhyme nor reason to their order.

I am not suggesting that an APD can be diagnosed from spelling samples. Nor am I suggesting that every child with poor invented or regular spelling abilities, even if their errors seem to be consistent with acoustic confusions, has a speech-sound-based APD. I am merely illustrating the manner in which an APD may affect spelling abilities and how the nature of the child's spelling abilities may shed some light on the nature of the underlying deficit. Spelling difficulties such as those discussed in this section represent merely one piece of the overall puzzle.

Spelling relies, at least in part, on hearing the sounds of speech correctly and, then, relating those speech sounds to orthographic symbols on a page. If a child has inadequate speech-sound, or *phonological,* representation in the brain, learning the letters of the alphabet and applying this knowledge to spelling may be much more difficult.

SEE SPOT RUN: AUDITORY PROCESSING AND READING

Spelling is only the first step in reading. To read fluently, we must be able to "sound out" the words on the page, a skill we refer to as *decoding* or *word-attack abilities.* Again, this skill requires us to associate a given speech sound with a given letter or combination of letters. To make it even more confusing, as we all know, some words in the English language are not spelled the way they sound. These words—which we refer to as irregular—must simply be memorized. This is called *sight word reading.* Different types of APD can affect the ability either to sound out or to recognize the gestalt pattern of words, leading to slow, laborious reading.

I would like to emphasize that the information presented in this section is not intended to be a complete, scientific treatment of reading and reading disorders. Not only is the topic of dyslexia, or reading disorders, vast, it is out of the scope both of this book and of my own area of specialty. Furthermore, there is some controversy as to the underlying nature of the various dyslexias, and what part auditory and visual abilities play in these disorders. Therefore, in this section, I will confine the discussion to those reading difficulties that have been shown to be associated with APD.

Phonological Awareness When we first begin to learn to read, each and every word must be sounded out using the sound-symbol associations we have learned along with our newfound knowledge of the ABC's. For example, we have all had the experience of helping a small child read the word *cat.* What do we do? We sound out each letter: C——A——T; then we bring the sounds a little closer together: C—A—T; then still closer: C–A–T; until, at some point, the child's eyes light up and he shrieks, "Cat!" This process, known as *sound blending,* is just one skill in a whole group of abilities that are collectively referred to as *phonological awareness abilities.*

Phonological awareness essentially means our ability to understand how speech sounds are used in words. Abilities that rely on phonological awareness include, but are not limited to, phonological manipulation, segmentation, and sound blending. An example of phonological manipulation is the ability to delete or alter the order of letters in a word and determine what the new word would be. Say *cat,* for example, without the *c* = *at.* Now add a *b* at the beginning = *bat.* Now, say the word backward = *tab.* Segmentation is the ability to separate out speech sounds in a word (for example, clap for each sound you hear in the word *black*—four claps: *b-l-a-ck*). Sound blending, as we have seen above, is the ability to take separate speech sounds and connect them in one meaningful utterance. Many tests that assess phonological awareness skills use activities similar to these examples.

Difficulties in phonological awareness may be indicative of an APD. However, these tasks require far more than just auditory processing. In the case of phonological manipulation, the child must, first, be able to remember and follow rather complex directions. Second, the child must certainly have a good representation of each speech sound—the *c* and *b* sounds in the case of *cat* and *bat*—in his brain and must be able to relate that representation to the letter or letters that are named. Third, the child must be able to segment the word *cat* into at least the *c* portion and the *at* portion. Finally, the child must be able to substitute the *b* sound for the *c* sound, then blend it all back together again to form the word *bat*. To say the word backward (*tab*), the child must be able to do all of the above tasks all over again and *then* resequence the whole thing in reverse order!

Amazing how difficult a seemingly simple task can be when you analyze each step, isn't it?

The sound-segmentation activity described above requires not only that the child have good phonological representations of each sound— requiring him to be able to hear each individual sound as a separate, distinct acoustic event—but also that he can demonstrate these distinct events through a completely different modality, such as motor skills or clapping. Likewise, sound blending, a task we use frequently when first learning how to sound out words, requires us to be able both to hear each separate speech sound and to know which sound corresponds to which letter(s) of the alphabet.

Certainly, difficulties with the phonological representation of speech sounds such as those found in APD may affect a child's ability to perform phonological awareness activities; however, so might a deficit in attention, memory, organizational skills necessary for sequencing the response, and a host of other factors. Therefore, although formal assessment of phonological awareness abilities may provide insight into whether a child may have an APD, it certainly does not provide a definitive answer.

Illustrating this point is a recent auditory processing consultation of mine on a seven-year-old boy with severe learning, including reading, difficulties. When an evaluation indicated that Karl had significant difficulties with phonological awareness as measured by a common test tool, his teacher suspected a possible APD. After reading these test results, I saw that Karl did, indeed, appear to have great difficulty with each and every phonological awareness skill assessed. However, when I delved deeper into the accompanying description of Karl's other difficulties, as well as the description of his performance during this specific testing, I began to question whether an APD was the likely culprit in this boy's learning disability.

Karl did have difficulty with phonological segmentation. However, his music teacher reported that he was unable to clap or march in rhythm and that he was frequently unable to coordinate his clapping movements at all. Because the segmentation activity required a clapping response, his poor performance on this task might have been due to difficulty in the motor output, not the segmentation itself.

Further insight came when I realized that Karl not only had difficulty manipulating the order of speech sounds in words, but that he also had trouble organizing colored blocks into groups or related pictures into categories. He was not able to place pictures in the appropriate order to tell a story.

Finally, and possibly most revealing, not only was Karl unable to associate speech sounds with letters of the alphabet, but he couldn't identify many of the letters of the alphabet at all. He was also inconsistent in his identification of numbers or colors.

All of this information led me to suspect that Karl's "phonological awareness" difficulties were probably not truly phonological at all, but reflected the difficulties he had with various aspects of the tasks in the testing—tasks that crossed a wide range of skills and raised suspicion of a more global, higher-level cognitive disorder.

As Karl's example illustrates, it is important to analyze the task demands, not just the outcome or final score, of any test tool. Only then can we begin to identify the underlying reasons for a child's difficulties. We must avoid the temptation of merely ascribing the overall test score to difficulties in the specific area the test tool is assumed to measure.

Sight-Word Reading   We learn to read by painstakingly sounding out each letter of each word and blending them together to form meaningful wholes. But, as time goes on, we become more familiar with the task and begin to rely less and less on sounding out the words. We begin to automatically recognize the overall pattern of the most frequently encountered words, an ability that is referred to as sight word reading. If you are a good reader, you intuitively know this. As you are reading these words on the page, your eyes fly along the lines rapidly and you only stop to sound out a word when it is unfamiliar to you. The familiar words do not require the same type of phonological attack skills that unfamiliar words require. Indeed, what was once so difficult and time-consuming now seems virtually effortless; that is, unless you encounter new, unfamiliar words or difficult language that is outside of your normal realm of experience. In these situations, the fluid progression of your eyes across the page stutters to a stop, you back up, and you instinctively fall back on your earliest experiences with reading: sounding out the words or sentences, in your mind or sometimes even aloud, to try to make sense of the sequence of letters or words on the page. Even an accomplished reader may automatically and unconsciously call forth these earlier, phonological-based word attack skills in these circumstances.

The transition from word-attack to sight-word reading is a developmental process. For example, my fourth-grade son has a list of "no excuse" words supplied by his teacher. These are words that children should be able to recognize (and spell) automatically by the fourth grade—or that should be within the child's *sight-word vocabulary* by this age. They include frequently encountered words such as *always, because, been, have, know, long, new, small, together, too, two, to, under, well, would,* and so on. Many, many words would be expected to be a part of the child's sight word vocabulary by the fourth grade.

On the other hand, some words must be learned as sight words from the very beginning because they do not follow normal phonological patterns and, therefore, cannot really be sounded out. These *irregular* words, such as *subtle, phlegm, psychic,* and *soiree,* just to name a few, must simply be memorized to be recognized from our very first encounter with them.

Dysfunction in different parts of the brain can affect our word attack or sight word reading abilities selectively. For example, damage or dysfunction in the language-dominant (usually left) temporal lobe may impair word attack abilities, primarily because this portion of the brain assumes the greatest responsibility for speech-sound processing and phonological representation. Furthermore, the left hemisphere has been linked to the ability to analyze wholes into their constituent parts, something that is certainly required when one considers phonological awareness activities. Therefore, left-hemisphere dysfunction can be considered generally to impair the *sound* portion of sound-symbol association.

Conversely, dysfunction in the right hemisphere of the brain has been shown to affect the ability to engage in part-to-whole synthesis, or *gestalt patterning.* Disorders of the right hemisphere can have an impact on the *symbol* portion of sound-symbol association, particularly as relates to the symbol formed by the combination of letters on the page. As a result, sight word abilities may be affected significantly by right-hemisphere dysfunction.

Finally, disorders in the portion of the brain that connects the two hemispheres—the corpus callosum and related structures—can impair the *association* aspect of sound-symbol association. In these disorders, the problem can neither be identified precisely as either word attack or sight word difficulties, but rather as a generalized difficulty affecting both types of abilities.

In the children referred to me for auditory processing evaluation, one of the most frequent academic complaints is difficulty with reading or spelling. One of my first questions is, what is the specific nature of the reading difficulties? Are word attack abilities intact, whereas sight word abilities are not? Is the reverse true? Does this appear to be a visual-based disorder in which the child transposes or reverses the order of letters in words, or even the letters themselves? Do visual interventions frequently employed in dyslexia, such as the use of colored filters on the page, have any effect on the child's reading ability? Have the child's phonological awareness abilities been assessed, and if so, were specific difficulties noted?

The answers to these questions shed light on whether the child's reading difficulty may stem from a problem in auditory processing. In addition, the nature of the child's reading difficulties may provide an insight into the possible site of dysfunction in the brain—something that may ultimately become very important when we are attempting to determine how an APD may be affecting a child's ability to learn, and the direction that management of the child's disorder should take.

Although not all reading disorders stem from auditory processing problems and not all cases of APD involve reading difficulties, the ability to read certainly involves an auditory component. Furthermore, certain types of APD are associated with certain types of difficulties in reading. That is, speech-sound-based APD is most often associated with word attack and phonological awareness difficulties, whereas sight word problems frequently accompany right-hemisphere-based APD. Finally, general difficulties in associating the sound with the symbol can occur in APD involving interhemispheric integration, or communication between the two hemispheres of the brain.

Word-Attack versus Sight-Word Abilities Following are some tips on how to separate word attack abilities from sight-word abilities in a child with reading difficulties. This information is not intended to substitute for a complete reading evaluation by a specialist in such disorders, nor is it intended to be diagnostic in nature. This information merely serves as a general guide to assist in understanding the nature and characteristics of a child's reading difficulties.

- Word-attack abilities: To gain a general idea of the child's ability to associate speech sounds with letters of the alphabet in decoding words, give the child a list of nonsense words—words that do not mean anything in our language, but that would be pronounced similarly if not identically by most readers—and have the child read them aloud. Try to use a variety of letters in each "word," and make the words only as long as is appropriate for the child's age. Because these nonsense words are not actually part of our language, children cannot rely on sight-word abilities to read them. Instead, good phonological awareness abilities are required. For example:

GORT
GLUMT
FRACK
CRATINATE
TIMPOT
EBNIG
FRIDIT
SIGNAP
CAGNIGAR

- Sight-word abilities: To obtain a general index of the child's sight word abilities, choose words that a child of his age should be able to recognize automatically but that don't necessarily rely on the ability to sound out phonologically. You should be able to get a grade-by-grade list of "no excuse" words from the child's teacher or from grade-level reading books available at the library or bookstore. Ask the child to read the words aloud—he should be able to do so rather quickly and automatically, without relying on phonological word-attack strategies.

- Have the child read a favorite book aloud. Note the words with which she has difficulty and ask yourself the following questions:

  1. Does she automatically read the easy, familiar words such as *to, and, the, with,* and so on, but bog down much more than would be expected when confronted with a new, unfamiliar word that must be sounded out? If so, word-attack difficulties may be the culprit.

  2. Does she attempt to attack even the familiar, frequent words using a phonological strategy every time they appear, ultimately succeeding at sounding them out? If so, sight-word reading may be difficult for her.

  3. If one word is unfamiliar at the beginning of the book, but appears again and again throughout, does her ability to read this word become more automatic each time it is presented, so that, by the end of the book, she recognizes the pattern more quickly than she did at the beginning? If so, it is likely that she is adding this word to her sight-word vocabulary appropriately.

  4. If one phonological strategy, such as the use of rhyming words in which the first letter is different, is used throughout the book, does the child catch on to this and begin to apply appropriate word-attack strategies to the beginning letters of each new word? If so, her word-attack skills are emerging. Note: Dr. Seuss books, such as *Cat in the Hat* or *Hop on Pop,* are particularly useful for this activity.

Reading disorders may arise from auditory processing difficulties or from many other factors. When reading problems are associated with an APD, an analysis of the underlying nature of the reading disorder can help us understand the relationship between the APD and the reading disorder and provide guidance for the development of intervention strategies that will directly address the child's difficulties. Finally, when a child (or adult) is coping with an APD that impacts reading, so much time and effort may be spent trying to decode each letter, each word, that, by the end of the sentence, the reader has forgotten what the sentence is about. As a result, reading comprehension can be affected by APD, as well.

THERE'S A BATHROOM ON THE RIGHT: AUDITORY PROCESSING AND RECEPTIVE LANGUAGE

In Creedence Clearwater Revival's song "Bad Moon Rising," there is a stanza that reads: "There's a bad moon on the rise." For years, I struggled to make sense of this song because I thought they said, "There's a bathroom on the right." This demonstrates how a problem in processing auditory information can impact the ability to understand what is being said. In this example, my own difficulty discriminating the words rendered me unable to grasp the meaning or context of the song. This is in contrast to when the language itself makes no sense even if every word is heard clearly—as in, for example, the Beatles' "I Am the Walrus" or Lewis Carroll's "Jabberwocky."

The Creedence example may be regarded as analogous to an APD that affects the clarity of the communication and, thus, garbles the message heard. The Beatles example, on the other hand, might be analogous to a true receptive language disorder in which the difficulty lies not with the clarity of the signal or, indeed, any input issue at all. Instead, the ability to grasp the meaning of the message is affected on a higher linguistic level. In other words, even if you heard and understood the meaning of each word of "I Am the Walrus," you would still have no idea what the song means because the language makes no sense.

It is very difficult to draw a line that cleanly delineates the point at which auditory processing leaves off and language begins, even though many in my own and related fields would like to do so. Indeed, as I often tell students in my neuroanatomy courses, I have seen a lot of brains, but I have yet to see one that is color-coded, with a clear demarcation between auditory and language areas, as they appear in textbooks. The difficulty in separating auditory processing from language may best be illustrated by the following two examples.

Harold was sixty-five years old. He was a professor of English at an East Coast university and had been a prolific writer and speaker. Then, one Saturday morning, he was sitting at his dining room table, drinking his coffee. His wife later explained, "A funny look came over his face, hard to describe, not pain exactly but more like confusion. He opened his mouth as though he was going to say something. Then he just fell to the floor." The paramedics were called and Harold was rushed to the hospital, where it was determined that he had suffered a massive stroke affecting the left hemisphere of his brain.

Harold spent several days in the intensive care unit. At first, his prognosis was guarded and his condition was touch and go. When he regained consciousness, it was apparent that he had lost many of his motor skills for the right side of his body, including his face, arm, and leg. He had great difficulty expressing himself, to the point that he would become frustrated and clench his good fist, sometimes banging it against the bed over and over in his agitation. He also couldn't write down his thoughts, but not because of his motor difficulties. Although Harold, a right-handed man, was now unable to hold a pencil in his right hand, he could not form the language necessary to write what he wanted to say even using his left hand. Harold did appear to understand relatively well, although he became somewhat confused if the information presented was very long or complex. And even though Harold seemed unable to produce speech spontaneously, he was able to repeat words easily. He had more difficulty with the repetition of sentences, however, just as he had more difficulty understanding complex information or instructions.

Over time, Harold's condition stabilized, and eventually he went home. Beginning in the hospital and continuing for many months, Harold received physical therapy to improve his right-sided motor skills as well as speech-language therapy to assist him with speaking and writing. His comprehension of language—both verbal and written—has improved markedly, and he rarely demonstrates difficulty understanding any but the most complex of messages.

However, Harold continues to have great difficulty choosing the right words with which to express himself—what we call *word retrieval abilities.* He often goes around and around the topic rather than saying the word itself, a strategy known as circumlocution. When I first met Harold, he told me how he and his wife lived in a house on a large plot of forest land, and loved to bird-watch. He even had a condor on his property that he spied occasionally. However, forced by his stroke to use bits and pieces of broken language, Harold was unable to remember the precise name for the bird. Instead, he said, "Black, you know. Rare, very rare, you know. Big and black. Big and rare, you know. Magnificent, oh, magnificent, you know." Harold had by this point come to terms with his language difficulties and was patient with me as I tried to figure out what he was talking about, even demonstrating his characteristic sense of humor through his laughter and the twinkle in his eye at my ignorance about birds.

This went on for several minutes. Harold never got frustrated—instead, he seemed to be enjoying himself, having a bit of fun at my own rising frustration as I began to name every bird I could think of. He laughed aloud when I said "Pigeon?" and even I had to acknowledge that this was a pretty stupid guess. Finally, in a rare burst of insight, I offered timidly, "Condor?" Harold immediately clapped his hands together, then pointed at me. "Condor!" he shouted, laughing as he patted me on the back. I felt so proud of myself for figuring out the puzzle, and Harold was proud of me, too, nodding enthusiastically as he exclaimed, "Good, yes, good! Condor. Magnificent, you know! Good." Somehow our roles had reversed. It never seemed to occur to either of us that my lack of understanding was due to Harold's communication disorder.

Once the bird puzzle was solved, I administered several behavioral tests of central auditory processing to see how his stroke had affected his performance on these tasks. This was possible because of Harold's preserved ability to repeat words and sentences, despite his difficulty in generating spontaneous speech and retrieving words on his own. My testing showed a pattern that was consistent with an APD—for example, he had difficulty in all of the dichotic listening tasks, with relatively greater difficulty repeating the information presented to the right ear. This finding was precisely what would be expected considering Harold's left-hemisphere damage. His speech-sound processing skills, his ability to fill in missing pieces of the message (auditory closure skills), and other auditory abilities were just fine in comparison.

So, my auditory processing tests were clearly indicative of a left-hemisphere-based APD that did not, however, affect speech-sound processing or auditory closure skills. Nevertheless, I don't feel that it would be accurate to state that Harold's difficulty lies in auditory processing per se. Certainly, his performance on my tests showed that these behavioral measures are able to identify left-hemisphere damage. But despite the finding of abnormalities on my testing, Harold's difficulty clearly lies in that higher-level language area—especially as his expressive writing skills are affected, as well—rather than in specific auditory areas. Oh, he has some problems understanding especially complex messages, as I've already pointed out, but this is not his primary, nor even one of his primary, presenting complaints.

Harold's diagnosis is language disorder. Specifically, Harold exhibits a common consequence of stroke: *aphasia*. Aphasia can take many forms; sometimes the ability to understand is impaired although speech production may be preserved. Other forms may have exactly the opposite effect. Some may affect functioning in both receptive and expressive domains. Sometimes reading and writing are affected, but sometimes not. Different types are associated with damage in different portions of the language dominant hemisphere. In short, we refer to these disorders not as a single entity, but rather in the plural—the aphasias—and specify which type we are referring to. In Harold's case, aphasia is certainly a far more appropriate label than APD.

Let's consider a different case—that of a young, school-aged girl who exhibits behavioral symptoms somewhat similar to those exhibited by Harold and, indeed, whose performance on behavioral auditory processing tests was identical to that of Harold, but for whom the label APD might be more appropriate.

Tracy was referred to me for a central auditory evaluation when she was in the third grade. Although her spelling and reading skills were age appropriate, her reading comprehension was not always up to par. Of primary concern, though, was Tracy's difficulty understanding information that was presented to her verbally. She had a difficult time following directions, especially directions involving multiple steps, such as "Take out your math book and a sheet of paper, turn to page thirteen, and complete problems one through six." Once she understood what was expected of her, she was able to complete the task. The hard part was getting her to understand the directions in the first place.

Similarly, Tracy frequently became confused when concepts were explained in particularly complex language or when the passive voice (e.g., "The ball was hit by the girl") was used. This difficulty led to poor grades in subjects such as science and social studies. Her receptive vocabulary—the number and type of words she was able to understand and identify—was within the normal range for her age, as were her expressive vocabulary abilities. She did, however, exhibit some mild word retrieval problems leading her to circumlocute occasionally. When shown a picture of a picnic table, Tracy might initially describe what it was used for ("You eat lunch on it outside") rather than naming it. She was, however, usually able to come up with the correct label eventually. Her hearing sensitivity was normal in both ears, despite her having had frequent ear infections as an infant and toddler. Phonological analysis skills were well developed, and she was able to discriminate easily among speech sounds, even those that sound very similar acoustically.

But Tracy's brain seemed to have a short circuit somewhere between the hearing of the speech sounds and the understanding of what the communication meant. Further, there did not appear to be any obvious reason why this bright child, who was easily able to pay attention to a task and appeared to be making a real effort, was having such comprehension difficulties.

When I tested Tracy, I found the same pattern of results as I had previously found with Harold. That is, Tracy had difficulty with dichotically presented information, particularly in her right ear, that led me to suspect left-hemisphere involvement. Like Harold, Tracy's auditory closure and phonological representation abilities, as measured by her ability to fill in the missing portions of a message and discriminate among similar-sounding words, appeared to be fine. Her right-hemisphere-based and interhemispheric auditory skills also seemed to be normal.

It appeared that Tracy did indeed exhibit an APD that was affecting her comprehension abilities, especially for complex information. She had done relatively well in her earlier elementary school grades. Her auditory deficit didn't really appear until the information presented in class became more linguistically complex, which usually happens at about the third-grade level. Based upon my pattern of test results, I felt that Tracy's difficulties lay not in the primary auditory areas of the brain where speech-sound representation takes place, but in those areas of the brain in which speech sounds and meaning come together—the *auditory association cortex*. These findings helped us to design an auditory-based management program that addressed Tracy's difficulty comprehending spoken language.

Why is it that I felt more comfortable applying the label APD to Tracy and not to Harold, even though both performed in precisely the same manner on behavioral tests of auditory processing? Was APD an appropriate label, or would the more accurate term perhaps be *receptive childhood aphasia*—a term that was once used to describe her type of difficulties?

There are no easy answers to these questions. Certainly, from a purely descriptive perspective, Harold's difficulties present themselves as more "language-like" in nature, whereas Tracy's problems appear to be more "auditory-like" in nature. That is, Harold has difficulty understanding only the most complex of messages, and his primary problem is in finding the right words to express himself. Tracy, on the other hand, has difficulty grasping the meaning of far less complex messages and behaves almost as if she can't hear what is being said at times. Also, the ways in which their disorders affect their daily lives differ, leading to very different management strategies for each. In Harold's case, his occasional difficulty understanding particularly complex language was a mild annoyance requiring no specific intervention. In Tracy's case, however, specific therapy was indicated to address her comprehension difficulties, which were far more apparent with spoken than with written language. But this distinction between "language-like" and "auditory-like" is extremely fuzzy and involves subtle judgments, not scientific distinctions.

That hearing, auditory processing, and language are inextricably intertwined is obvious when one considers the impact hearing disorders or sensory deprivation have on the development of language. At one point in our history, language researchers were vehemently involved in the "nature versus nurture" debate. The nature proponents stated that our development of language is an innate, biologically wired capability that is simply an evolutionary aspect of being human. The nurture proponents, on the other hand, argued that it is our exposure to and experience with language, gleaned from interactions with other humans, that ultimately guides our linguistic aptitude.

In time, we realized that neither the nature nor the nurture explanation fully accounted for the marvelous complexity of this dance of sound and meaning that we refer to as language. Rather, research into the neurophysiologic bases of language indicates that, indeed, we are biologically prewired with the fundamental capability to learn to understand and speak any of the myriad languages of the world. However, this innate wiring is not enough. Research into neuroplasticity—or the ability of the brain to change with stimulation and learning or the lack thereof—has definitively proven that it is our experience with linguistic input that will ultimately determine which brain pathways are pruned away like the unnecessary branches of a tree and which will form strong connections among various brain structures and determine our ability to use and comprehend language.

The importance of language abilities in helping to overcome APD deserves some attention. A disorder in the "input" system that disrupts the clarity of what is heard can affect what is ultimately understood, but the person's *top-down* cognitive and linguistic abilities are just as important in compensating for a deficit at a lower, *bottom-up,* input level. The better a person's language skills, the more able he will be to compensate for an auditory processing deficit, as appeared to be the case with Harold.

Auditory Closure   One example of the use of higher-order language to assist in bottom-up auditory processing is *auditory closure,* the ability to fill in missing pieces of a message. If you have ever assembled a jigsaw puzzle, you know it is much easier if you have a picture to refer to or if you know what the final assembly is supposed to represent. A similar principle applies to auditory closure abilities. It is far easier to fill in the missing pieces of a message when you have a general idea of what the message is and a good vocabulary from which to choose likely candidates.

For example, suppose you are listening to a lecture on a topic of interest to you: volcanoes. You are seated near the back of the auditorium, directly behind a group of teenagers discussing the exciting events of the latest school dance. To make matters worse, the auditorium's acoustics are not the best. You hear the speaker say something about "Helens." Now, there are many Helens he could be referring to. Perhaps his wife is named Helen. Or perhaps he has suddenly diverted from the topic and begun talking about Helen of Troy. However, your familiarity with the topic and vocabulary of volcanoes is likely to lead you to a more logical interpretation: he is probably discussing Mount St. Helens. In this way, you are able to pick up the thread of the lecture once again even though you missed some of the message. You have relied on your higher-level language, vocabulary, and knowledge of the context to compensate for what your auditory system failed to pick up.

That we automatically fill in missing pieces of a word or message based on our language ability, vocabulary, and knowledge of the context has been demonstrated by experiments in which segments of words have been excised—literally taken out—and replaced with a cough or other nonspeech sound. Normal listeners not only automatically fill in the missing segment, but they are completely unaware that anything was missing at all. This filling-in seems to be such an automatic process that we engage in on a daily basis, a process that appears to be mediated by the brain itself, and one that we simply are not aware of in most situations. However, individuals with certain types of APD, language, or cognitive disorders, or who are unfamiliar with the vocabulary or context, are consciously aware of the excision and are frequently unable to fill in the missing segment—or "close" on the word. Therefore, the degree to which we are able to use our vocabulary, language, knowledge of context, and other factors directly relates to our perception, even at its most basic level.

I have often wondered whether the fundamental difference in the way Harold's and Tracy's deficits manifested themselves was not due, at least in part, to Harold's having had higher-level language abilities before his stroke, whereas Tracy's language abilities had not developed to a level at which she could depend on them to assist with her APD. Harold had a greater store of knowledge and vocabulary upon which to draw to understand communication. Tracy's store was minimal.

We shouldn't conclude that all language disorders arise from APD.

Nor should we assume that all forms of APD necessarily affect language abilities. Rather, auditory processing and language are interdependent, entwined in a complicated dance of sound and meaning that cannot be unraveled.

THE RAIN IN SPAIN: AUDITORY PROCESSING AND SPEECH PRODUCTION

How we speak is highly dependent on what we hear. When an infant is born, she has the innate ability to produce all of the sounds of any language of the world. The particular language that is heard, however, and the speech sounds used in that language, will determine what the infant is able to articulate. One of the most familiar examples of this is the difficulty Japanese speakers have with the *l* sound. Because this sound does not occur in the Japanese language, they have little experience hearing it and, therefore, cannot produce it, either. Instead, they substitute the closest-sounding phoneme from their language—*r*—in English words. There have been many studies of the link between nonnative speech sound perception and production. These studies have shown that, for example, native Japanese listeners are also unable to discriminate between *r* and *l* when they hear exemplars of the two phonemes. Following specific auditory training in perceiving and discriminating these speech contrasts, however, their ability to produce the *l* sound also shows a dramatic improvement. Thus, production mirrors perception.

The difficulty Japanese listeners have in producing the *l* sound is not attributed to motor control of the mouth—or oral-motor difficulties. To appreciate this distinction, consider the following example: I can easily hear the difference between the Spanish *r,* as in the word for "but"—*pero*—and the *rr* as in the word for "dog"—*perro.* I cannot, however, produce the difference because I cannot "roll my tongue" as is required in the word *perro.* As a result, I am far better at understanding Spanish than I am at producing it, for a purely oral-motor reason.

In contrast to this, there are many sounds in many languages that I can neither perceive nor produce, like the Japanese listeners discussed earlier. An excellent example would be the vocalic clicks used in some African languages. To the native speakers of these languages, each type of click is clearly different and carries a different meaning. To me, however, they are all just clicks—I can hear them, but I can neither discriminate among them nor produce them.

Articulation errors in children are common. They are to be expected up until as late as age seven. A normally developing young child may substitute a number of phonemes in their speech, all of which are perfectly normal developmentally. However, this does not mean that the child can't hear the difference between the phonemes they are unable to produce. A three-year-old child may, for example, say, "Mommy, I have to go to the bafroom." The substitution of *f* for *th* is common at this age and is considered normal. But if you mirror his production—"You have to go to the bafroom?"—he will probably correct you immediately: "No, Mommy. I have to go to the bafroom." He is clearly telling you that he can perceive the difference between the *f* and *th* sounds, but simply cannot produce the *th* sound.

Because certain speech sounds are more difficult to discriminate than others, the articulation errors made by a child can provide us with some information regarding the manner in which he hears the sounds of speech. In addition, articulation errors that are not considered typical of normally developing children or that appear to be auditory may be a key red flag of an auditory processing difficulty.

Speech-Sound Production It's important to understand this concept, so let's take a look at the normal development of speech-sound production in English-speaking children. This information was taken from the work completed in the 1950s by Mildred Templin and outlined in her classic book, *Certain Language Skills in Children*.

- By age three, a child should be able to produce most of the sounds of English. Although the child may still make some articulation errors, his speech should be intelligible to strangers. Speech sounds that are acquired by age three include *m, n, ng, p, f, h,* and *w.*

- By the age of three and a half, the *y* sound should be acquired (as in *y*es).

- By age four, sounds such as *k, b, d, g,* and *r* should be produced accurately. More difficult sounds, such as *s, sh,* and *ch,* may not be acquired until slightly later, at the age of approximately four and a half.

- By age six, the child should be able to produce *t, v, l,* and *th* (as in ba*th*room).

- The most difficult sounds of English, which may not be acquired until age seven, include *z, zh* (as in measure), *th* (as in fa*th*er), and *j.*

Other general principles that apply to normal speech development include the use of "frozen phrases" in earlier years. Examples of frozen phrases include *lmno* when saying the alphabet and utterances such as "Where'ditgo?" In these examples, the child is not completely aware of the demarcation between each portion of the utterance. For example, if you try to get a small child to say the alphabet slowly (which may be difficult, as she is more apt to try to sing it), you will find that the child segments the alphabet in the way she is accustomed to doing in the song. Therefore, *lmno* becomes one letter of the alphabet. (Try singing the alphabet song yourself. LMNO sound as if they are all one letter, don't they?) Similarly, when the child asks, "Where'ditgo?" she is not aware of the phonological distinctions within and between the words: "Where did it go?" Rather, she is using one frozen phrase to express the rather complex concept "It was here a minute ago, and now it's gone. Where did it go?"

Using these general guideposts, we can begin to determine the underlying nature of a child's speech-production difficulties. Certainly, articulation errors that persist long after the normal age of acquisition of speech sounds suggest that a child may not be hearing the sounds of speech clearly. However, articulation errors may also arise from errors in motor planning or from difficulty with coordinating the various parts of the speech mechanism—the mouth, tongue, lips, teeth, and so on—to produce a word correctly.

Perhaps another audience participation experiment is in order here. Say aloud the sounds *d* and *g*, paying careful attention to what structures in your mouth are coming into contact with each other during the production of each. With *d*, your tongue lightly taps the ridge just behind your front teeth. With *g*, on the other hand, the very back of your tongue rises and taps the back portion of the top of your mouth, or your palate. D is produced toward the front of the mouth and *g* is produced toward the back of the mouth.

We have seen that the auditory distinction between the *d* and *g* is slight; they sound quite similar to one another. Articulation errors in which these sounds are confused may be due to difficulties in hearing these very subtle differences. On the other hand, if the child is younger than four, the same articulation errors may be developmental in nature—that is, due to accidentally producing the *g* like a *d* (a process known as *fronting*) or, conversely, producing a *d* like a *g* (*backing*). Even in an older child, the same articulation errors could be due either to oral-motor issues or to auditory issues.

For this reason, it is critical that someone with a knowledge of normal and disordered speech-sound production be enlisted in any assessment of speech-sound production problems. The professional uniquely qualified and certified to address such issues is the speech-language pathologist, and his or her involvement in the analysis of speech-production disorders in children is absolutely imperative when we are attempting to determine whether articulation errors may be due to an underlying difficulty in auditory processing. Therefore, as in all of the situations described in this chapter, although an APD may lead to articulation deficits, not all articulation deficits are due to APD.

That having been said, there is no doubt that auditory processing problems can affect speech production at the basic speech-sound level, or at the level of connected speech and expression of linguistic concepts. Remember Clay, the four-year-old nonverbal boy? Clay's speech was unintelligible even to his mother long after the age at which it should have been understandable to strangers, notwithstanding a few developmental articulation errors. No oral-motor or other difficulty could possibly account for this unintelligibility, yet the types of errors he made in speech production were not typical of normally developing children. Still, he was able to produce many sounds when he could see the mechanism of the articulation.

Because I work in a university speech and hearing clinic, I interact daily with speech-language pathology colleagues in the department. Frequently, we team together to attempt to unravel the speech and language difficulties of the children who come to us for assistance. We have seen many children like Clay, children for whom a "speech-based" explanation seems unlikely but who, nevertheless, are unable to speak intelligibly. In many of these cases, APD is suspected, and in some situations—such as Clay's—we can confirm the presence of an auditory processing deficit. Our interdisciplinary collaboration allows us to focus our management and intervention directly on the underlying nature of each child's disorder. In Clay's case, we decided to focus on both perception and production in tandem so that we were able to improve both his auditory and speech abilities. Focusing on Clay's speech and language alone had been minimally effective in remediating his disorder. Auditory training alone probably wouldn't have had much of an impact, either. Clay's remarkable and rapid progress was the result of carefully planned teamwork between professionals and students in speech-language pathology and audiology who were able to design a program that addressed, intensively, both auditory processing and speech production simultaneously.

What we say and how we say it are closely tied to what we hear. APD and speech-production disorders may go hand-in-hand. By analyzing the type of speech-production errors a child makes, and comparing these to typical developmental errors or errors that arise from difficulties in planning or executing oral movements, we can begin to determine whether a young child may be exhibiting an APD that is affecting his or her speech production. To do this, however, requires interdisciplinary interaction between professionals knowledgeable about speech and language disorders and those who work with APD.

HOW LONG IS THE DIVING BOARD? AUDITORY PROCESSING AND PROBLEM-SOLVING

My oldest brother once characterized college algebra word problems as follows: "The swimming pool is ten feet by fifteen feet. The depth of the water is eight feet in the deep end and three feet in the shallow end. When siphoning the water for cleaning, a two-inch tube can drain the water at a rate of two gallons per minute. How long is the diving board?"

Some of the children referred to me for auditory processing assessment or consultation have difficulties with mathematics. Others have excellent mathematics ability but poor achievement in more language-based subjects such as social studies and English. Although math is not typically considered a "verbal" skill (it does not seem to rely on auditory or language abilities), it is important to take a detailed look at the problems of a child or adult who has "difficulties with math."

In the college algebra problem, language clearly plays a critical role. The student must be able to read the problem or to hear it if it is presented verbally. All of the relevant information must be present. He must understand the words used and the concepts involved and remember them. He must be able to identify which computations to apply and then sequence them appropriately. Finally, he must be able to perform those computations correctly to arrive at an accurate answer. This is a very different situation from a teacher's writing a problem on the board such as $13 + 84 = ?$

Many of the children with whom I work demonstrate little difficulty in straight arithmetic calculation using numbers only, but have great difficulty with verbally presented or written math word problems. Conversely, some people also have difficulty with the calculation itself, people such as Jason or, indeed, myself. For both of us, math calculation difficulties are part of an overall right-hemisphere-based dysfunction that also includes right-hemisphere auditory processing difficulties.

This distinction is important. We know that people with APD typically have greater difficulty with verbal or language-based subjects than with mathematics. However, I have seen this statement so overgeneralized that any child with poor grades in math is automatically excluded from consideration of a possible APD. To avoid making these overgeneralizations, we must take a careful look at the specific types of mathematics difficulty the child is exhibiting and consider this information in light of the additional information from other academic and related areas.

This distinction has led to some confusion and misunderstanding of intellectual test results by people who are not familiar with psychological cognitive testing. One of the most commonly used tests of cognitive ability, or IQ, is the Weschler Intelligence Scale for Children (WISC-III). From this test, three types of IQ scores can be calculated. The Performance IQ is an index of the child's nonverbal intellectual abilities, including visual-spatial skills, ability to assemble objects, picture sequencing skills, and similar activities. The Verbal IQ is an index of the child's ability to perform auditory- and language-based tasks. The Full Scale IQ is obtained by averaging the Performance and Verbal scores. In the WISC-III, the arithmetic subtest is included under the Verbal IQ scale. Although it might seem that arithmetic would be more appropriately considered under nonverbal intellectual abilities, the WISC-III requires the child to solve verbally presented arithmetic word problems. Therefore, this mathematics subtest is clearly a measure of verbal comprehension abilities in addition to math calculation abilities and, as such, is considered a measure of Verbal IQ.

My ten-year-old son recently brought home a page of word problems. One of them read as follows:

> *The fourth grade decided to raise funds by selling apples. They sold 33 apples on Sunday, 45 apples on Monday, and 106 apples on Tuesday. How many more apples did they sell on Tuesday than they sold on Sunday and Monday combined?*

Some key words in this exercise simply must be heard and understood if the child is to have any hope of solving the problem. For example, each number (33, 45, and 106) and their respective days (Sunday, Monday, Tuesday) are critical. Also critical are the words that relate to the mathematics calculation that will be required, such as *more* and *combined*. It really doesn't matter whether the child understands that this is a fund-raiser or that the kids are selling apples—this part is just extraneous information that isn't necessary for solving the problem.

If the child misses any of the critical components of this word problem, as a child with an APD might do—particularly if the problem is presented verbally—the answer will be inaccurate. But a child may arrive at an inaccurate answer for many reasons. He may not remember the information. He may have a difficult time planning and sequencing the steps required. Or maybe he doesn't understand what types of computations are required to address the "more" topic (subtraction) or the "combined" topic (addition). Finally, the child may be able to perform all of these steps perfectly well, but have difficulty with the calculation itself: $106 - (33 + 45) = ?$ But certainly, difficulty with perceiving and understanding the language of the overall problem and the critical components of the problem, such as may occur with an APD, will destroy the child's chance for success right at the outset.

When I see a child in whom an APD is suspected and I am told that he is failing math, I always ask about the specific nature of the math problems. Does he not catch the key components or understand the overall language of the problem? Does he become confused when trying to sequence his responses or choosing which computations to apply? Or does he, like me, get to the final stage only to have difficulty with the calculations themselves? Finally, if he is an older child, how does he fare with more visual-based, less language-based math skills such as those required in geometry? Many people with right-hemisphere-based dysfunction have difficulty with geometry because of the strong visual and calculation components. I then consider this information, as always, in light of the child's other academic and communicative complaints to determine whether his overall pattern of difficulties has a common, possibly auditory-based, link.

Math word problems are not the only type of problem-solving activities that can be affected by auditory processing deficits and related difficulties. Any problem-solving requires that the critical elements be identified before they can be acted on. The ability to identify the key words or main theme of a message may be difficult for many individuals with APD, especially those in which the right hemisphere is involved. Yet this ability is important for understanding communication.

When giving an assignment or delivering a lecture, a teacher may use more words than necessary. For example, she may say, "Okay, class, your assignment is to write a term paper. Now, don't complain. It only needs to be five pages long. I know that may seem like a lot right now, but you'll find it's much easier than you think once you start writing. You can pick any topic you want, as long as it has something to do with the American Revolution. You could write about Paul Revere's ride, or the first shots fired at North Bridge, or anything else that interests you. I really just want to see how well you can put your ideas down on paper. Let's see, this is Monday. If you hand the papers in by Wednesday, you'll have two days to complete the assignment. That should be plenty of time."

Here, the child with APD is faced with a problem to be solved. She is aware that an assignment has been given, and that she is expected to complete it on time. To solve this problem, she must separate the critical elements of the message from all of the extraneous language the teacher used. She must hear the number of pages (five), the topic (American Revolution), and the due date (Wednesday). She could ignore virtually everything else the teacher said and still successfully complete the assignment.

Solving problems of any kind relies on the fundamental principles of having all of the information, being able to manipulate the factors in one's mind, and arriving at a solution that must then be planned and carried out. If any step in this process is disrupted, our ability to problem-solve will be affected. This ability will most certainly suffer if we have difficulty obtaining all the information, as frequently happens when an individual has an APD. Moreover, when the problem is posed in a complex manner, with a lot of unnecessary language or difficult-to-understand wording, problem-solving will be affected even more dramatically when an individual has an APD. Therefore, although the ability to solve problems is not an auditory skill per se, it does rely, at least in part, on underlying auditory and language competencies.

MAKE NEW FRIENDS: AUDITORY PROCESSING AND SOCIALIZATION

Have you ever tried to join a conversation but, because you had missed some of what had been said, your contribution was off the topic? Unless you were with close friends or family (who would simply laugh and fill you in on what you had missed), it is likely that one of two things happened: either the others in the discussion politely ignored your input and went on as if you hadn't spoken or, even more mortifying, knowing glances were exchanged along with barely suppressed titters of laughter discreetly hidden behind cupped hands. Can you remember the feeling of embarrassment that flooded through you?

Now, can you imagine this situation occurring almost every time you try to converse?

We are social animals. Even before we learn our first real words, we babble and coo, shriek and blow raspberries, engaging in vocal play both for the sheer joy of hearing our own voices and for the wonderful experience of coaxing laughter and smiles from those around us. We need this interaction with others, crave it in the same way we crave food when we are hungry or water when we thirst. And for most of us, what we receive in return is so enjoyable that it encourages us to continue to communicate.

But to be an effective communicator, either on the playground or in the boardroom, we must be able to hear and understand what is being said. We must also be able to comprehend subtle exchanges, such as those involving sarcasm or humor, and to "read between the lines" to determine the hidden meanings underlying the words themselves. Different types of APD may affect each of these abilities in different ways. For the individual with APD, social communication is frequently a chore rather than a pleasure.

A child or adult who does not hear clearly, especially in noisy environments, may often misunderstand what is being said. As a result, his input into the conversation may be off-topic or inappropriate. When this occurs frequently, he may begin to be excluded from social groups, even laughed at for being "slow." Sometimes, the person with an APD may have other talents to fall back on—sports, music, art—and be able to carve a place for himself in the social world and to earn the respect of others based on these skills. However, even the talented individual with an APD may be ridiculed behind his back or to his face. Over time, individuals with APD may come to perceive themselves through others' eyes, to see themselves as others see them—as slow, dim, stupid, incompetent.

Although some people may persevere in the face of such discouragement, becoming the class clown or the good-natured dumb jock for the sake of being included in the social whirl, others may withdraw from social contact and self-isolate in an attempt to avoid embarrassment and ridicule. These people may, in defense, exclude themselves before others have a chance to exclude them. They may even behave antisocially and protest that they prefer to be alone.

Teenagers with APD may be loners or go to extremes to be part of a group, even if it requires acting against their own ethical or moral values. In the adolescents and teenagers I have worked with, I have seen a higher incidence of sexual promiscuity among those, especially girls, with APD. I have witnessed an extraordinarily high prevalence of APD in the juvenile delinquent population—teens incarcerated for gang behavior, truancy, and drug use. Although sociological research has clearly shown that many other family, economic, and peer-related factors may lead to these types of behaviors, certainly the inability to engage in socially appropriate interaction and communication with same-aged peers can be a predisposing element, as well. Furthermore, because poor social judgment and pragmatic language abilities frequently accompany right-hemisphere-based disorders, individuals with right-hemisphere APD may fare even worse than those for whom speech-sound processing is affected.

Adults with APD will frequently avoid situations in which they anticipate communication difficulties. Because an APD is usually more evident in noisy situations or where several people are talking at once, adults may avoid any environment like that, including malls, cocktail or dinner parties, and church socials. Over time, they, too, may become loners, preferring the safe isolation of their living rooms to the uncertain communicative environments of the outside world.

At home, APD can drive a wedge between loved ones. When one partner has an APD, the frustration of the other partner at constantly being misheard or misunderstood can lead to arguments that might never have arisen otherwise. Despite their best intentions, parents may berate the child with an APD for not doing what he is told, for not paying attention, for never listening when he is spoken to. In time, the child or adult with an APD may come to feel unloved, unworthy, unimportant, and a burden to his family.

APD often has a dramatic impact on a person's ability to engage in social communication. Although many of the people I see for central auditory evaluation or consultation are referred to me because of difficulties in academic areas such as reading or spelling, the social difficulties that accompany their APD are far and away the most distressing of their complaints. Although it is neither desirable nor recommended, we can get through life hiding a weakness in reading or spelling. Once we graduate from school, we can usually manage to avoid mathematics most of the time. As adults, we can simply refuse to play games such as Scrabble or cribbage, we can hire accountants to do the books, we can watch videos instead of losing ourselves in a novel. We can choose careers that do not rely on skills that we have difficulty with. Our weaknesses in these areas need not be broadcast to the world around us.

But we can neither hide nor run from the social communication difficulties that can accompany APD. We wear them like an ill-fitting coat, and they are apparent to anyone who looks carefully enough at us. Of all the difficulties that arise from auditory processing problems, those that impact our ability to interact with others strike the deepest, hurt the worst, most demean ourselves in our own eyes. Even if we ignore the potential effects APD may have on other aspects of language and learning, here is reason enough to emphasize early identification and management of auditory processing problems.

3

APD IN CHILDREN

A BABY IS BORN. We count fingers and toes, examine ears and nose and chin. Our heart swells with an almost indescribable wealth of love the first time that tiny hand closes around our finger, the first time those eyes open to peer curiously at our face, the little brow furrowed as if to say, "What strange and wondrous world have I suddenly ended up in?"

This new life is like a sponge, eager to fill himself with new experiences and sensations. Watch an infant closely during the first few weeks of life and you cannot help but notice that, when he is not sleeping, crying, or eating, a good deal of time is spent in "quiet wakefulness"—in which he simply lies back in his cradle and takes it all in. Although the baby appears to be doing nothing, his little brain is cataloging what he sees and hears and feels: the sound of his mother's voice, the texture of the blanket covering him, the contrasting lights and darks of the mobile spinning above his little head. He is learning, and new connections are being forged in his brain, connections that will form the basis of everything that is to come.

When a new object is placed before an infant, he will try to focus on it, sometimes frowning comically and crossing his eyes so that he can examine this strange new item. New sounds are cataloged, too—a loving voice comforts and calms, a sudden bark of a dog may startle. If the baby is born into a loud household, he quickly learns not to become too startled at the familiar shout of a sibling or a dog bark, although the sudden occurrence of either might still set him to crying. By listening to the voices and sounds around him, the baby begins to learn the basics of communication.

Auditory processing problems can appear at any point in life, but when APD occurs in infants and children, it can have a dramatic, often devastating, impact on learning, academic success, and even basic interaction with the world. This chapter contains key information regarding APD in children, including stages of normal speech and language development, red flags that an APD may be present in children of various ages, and ways in which APD may affect learning and communication in preschool, elementary school, middle and high school, or college.

SHAKE, RATTLE, AND ROLL: APD IN INFANTS AND TODDLERS

It is often difficult to know whether an APD was present at birth or occurred later in life. However, some cases of APD do appear very early in the life of the child, leading to problems in normal speech and language acquisition. When we consider APD in infants and toddlers, we must have an understanding of normal speech and language development so that potential problems or disorders can be detected as early as possible.

NORMAL SPEECH AND LANGUAGE IN THE INFANT AND TODDLER YEARS

It is important to consider the stages of normal speech and language in the infant and toddler years, as well as those factors that may place a child at risk for auditory and related problems. Unfortunately, we are not completely aware of all the risk factors that can lead to APD in children. Moreover, most hearing, speech/language, and auditory processing disorders occur without a clear cause. This, perhaps more than anything else, may be the most frustrating aspect of many disorders that affect listening, learning, and communication—the realization that we are often completely unable to pin down a precise reason for a child's difficulties. Nevertheless, the infant's early health, as well as the family history, should be considered when attempting to determine why a child may be having difficulties in some areas or, conversely, when attempting to predict which children may be at a higher risk for language, learning, or hearing problems.

The Joint Committee on Infant Hearing (JCIH), a group comprising audiologists, otologists (ear specialists), pediatricians, and deaf educators, among others, has worked hard over the years to identify what factors may lead to hearing loss in infants. The JCIH has also developed guidelines for early screening and follow-up of infants thought to be at risk and, most recently, for all infants. The group's primary focus has been the early identification of hearing loss or deafness in infants. However, the JCIH recommendations may also be applicable to APD and other hearing-related disorders because any factor that may place a child at high risk for ear-based auditory problems may, likewise, place the child at high risk for problems anywhere in the auditory system. Because the effects of APD frequently mimic the effects of hearing loss, it is important to rule out hearing loss at the earliest age possible.

The JCIH "Year 2000 Position Statement" identifies the following neonatal and early-childhood factors that may place an infant or toddler at risk for hearing loss:

- Any illness or condition that requires the baby to be admitted for forty-eight hours or more to a neonatal intensive care unit (NICU)

- Physical signs of any of the many syndromes known to be associated with hearing loss, such as Down's syndrome or Treacher-Collins syndrome

- History of permanent childhood hearing loss in the family

- Any visible abnormality of the head or face, including even mild deformations of the ear

- History of an infection in the mother during pregnancy such as rubella, herpes, toxoplasmosis, or cytomegalovirus (CMV)

- History of an infection in the baby after birth that may be associated with hearing loss, such as bacterial meningitis

- Infant conditions after birth such as severe jaundice (requiring blood transfusion) and breathing problems requiring the baby to be assisted by a ventilator or to be given oxygen

- Presence of any syndrome associated with hearing loss that worsens over time

- Presence of any neurological disorder that results in deterioration of motor or sensory function over time

- History of head trauma

- History of repeated or chronic ear infections with fluid in the middle ear for at least three months

- Any concern on the part of parents, caregivers, or others regarding hearing, speech, language, and/or developmental delay

Although these high-risk factors have been shown to be associated with hearing loss in infants and children, many of them can affect development and functioning across a wide variety of sensory and cognitive domains. A lack of oxygen at birth, for example, can cause a number of developmental and sensory difficulties, hearing loss being only one. These factors may be useful in determining which children may be at a greater risk for APD, although some may, with further research, prove not to be associated with APD at all. We simply have not yet identified the high-risk factors for APD. For example, although children with APD usually do not have a family history of permanent childhood sensorineural hearing loss, APD in many cases does seem to have some familial or genetic component. Many of the parents of children with APD report that they also had listening, language, or learning difficulties during childhood. Therefore, a family history of any type of hearing, language, or learning problems may be a high-risk factor for APD.

In the past, it was recommended that infants who had any of the risk factors identified by the JCIH be screened as early as possible for hearing loss, preferably before leaving the hospital.

Now, however, these recommendations have been extended to include all infants. This is because data collected over the years have shown that the high-risk registry fails to identify many, even most, children with hearing loss. In addition, many of the children with clear high-risk factors do not, indeed, end up with hearing loss at all. For this reason, we are now emphasizing the need for universal newborn hearing screening programs—or the screening of all babies born, whether high-risk or not, for early identification of hearing problems. The Newborn Hearing Screening and Intervention Act was passed by Congress in 1999, and the Children's Health Act of 2000, signed by President Clinton in May of 2000, extended the provisions of this act for another two years.

The ultimate goal of this act is to provide hearing screening services to all infants born in the United States. The act also provides for follow-up and early intervention for all infants or children identified with hearing loss. At the present time, many states have mandated and provided funding for universal hearing screening for all infants, although the federal act does not require that states mandate such programs. Other states are in the planning or development stages of similar programs, to be either voluntary or mandatory. Those states or areas that do not yet have universal hearing screening continue to screen the hearing of those infants identified by the JCIH register to be at risk.

Although this legislation marks a dramatic breakthrough in our ability to identify and treat hearing loss in very young children, a few critical distinctions must be made regarding APD.

Hearing versus Processing Passing a hearing screening or verification of normal hearing acuity does not mean that the child is *processing* what she hears adequately. The first step in attempting to determine why a child may have language or listening problems should be to rule out a hearing loss. This requires testing by an audiologist trained in pediatric audiology. It is important to realize, however, that such testing measures only whether the infant or child can *detect* sound. It makes no statement about whether the infant can discriminate among different sounds or can perceive or understand speech. The overall act of hearing and understanding what we hear includes the outer ear, middle ear, inner ear, auditory nerve, central auditory pathways, *and* the brain. A problem in any of these areas can affect the ability to hear or process sounds. The majority of children with APD exhibit completely normal hearing sensitivity as measured by standard audiologic tests. The finding of "normal hearing" by standard hearing tests refers only to *what* is heard, not *how* it is heard.

Limits of Newborn Hearing Screening The tests used for newborn hearing screening are physiologic screening tools and may miss many types of auditory disorders. Although we have been referring to newborn "hearing" screening, it should be understood that we are not actually testing the infant's hearing. In other words, these tests tell us if certain parts of the auditory system appear to be functioning properly, but they give us no information about whether the infant can actually detect and process sound. For example, otoacoustic emissions (OAEs)— the tool used in many hearing screening programs—test only the function of a portion of the inner ear. Therefore, OAEs will not detect problems in the auditory nerve or the central auditory pathways, even if these problems cause a hearing loss in the infant. A prime example of this type of condition is *auditory neuropathy,* a disorder of the auditory nerve that results in both hearing loss and severe auditory processing problems. When an infant has auditory neuropathy, OAEs are perfectly normal because the site of dysfunction is beyond the inner ear. Therefore, infants with auditory neuropathy will pass the newborn "hearing" screening if OAEs are used as the screening tool.

In contrast, the use of auditory electrophysiology screening tools, such as the *auditory brainstem response* (ABR), will be abnormal in cases of auditory neuropathy, but may also be abnormal for a host of other reasons related to neurological function that do not affect hearing itself. Or it may be, and most often is, completely normal in disorders in which the dysfunction is higher up in the brain, as is the case with the majority of auditory processing deficits. Therefore, ABR is not likely to identify most infants at risk for auditory processing problems.

Finally, both OAEs and the ABR will be affected by conditions of the outer and middle ear that are medically treatable, such as ear infections or fluid or debris in the ear as a result of birth. Therefore, some infants who fail hearing screening by OAEs or ABR will not have permanent hearing problems. In any case, neither of these screening tools tells us if the infant is actually hearing—or consciously perceiving—the sounds, nor do they tell us how the infant is processing the sounds that are heard. However, they do help identify those infants who may have hearing problems that need to be addressed.

Later-Onset Hearing Loss Passing a hearing screening at birth does not rule out hearing loss or other auditory problems that may occur during the first year of life or later. Some hearing losses are not present at birth. Instead, they appear sometime later and may get worse over time. For this reason, the JCIH recommendations include the presence of diseases or disorders associated with progressive hearing loss, as well as the presence of chronic ear infections that persist for more than three months. Any illness, injury, or other factor that may affect hearing and auditory processing during the first three years of life can have a significant impact on the child's language and learning abilities.

Limited Information Regarding High-Risk Factors for APD It is possible, even probable, that factors not included in the JCIH high-risk registry may lead to auditory processing problems. By and large, most of the high-risk factors for hearing loss identified by the JCIH represent pretty serious and obvious conditions in the newborn and young child. But most cases of APD are subtle and represent subtle dysfunction in the auditory system. Therefore, milder conditions that are not included in the list of high-risk indicators may lead to APD even though they may not affect hearing acuity itself.

When I first see a child for suspected hearing or auditory processing problems, I ask the parents a series of questions that delve into the baby's earliest history. These questions seek information about the pregnancy and the birth itself: Were there any complications? Did the mother have any illnesses or infections during pregnancy? Was the mother taking any medications during the pregnancy, particularly during the first trimester? Was the birth uncomplicated, or were there signs of fetal distress or other birth-related complications? I also ask about the baby's health immediately after the birth as well as about any pertinent medical and developmental history up to the time that I see the child. Parents need to have as much information as possible about the health and development of their child so that accurate information can be provided during a parent interview such as this. It is possible that even relatively innocuous complications or problems during the pregnancy or birth may place the child at a higher risk for processing problems such as APD.

When a baby is born, the delivery room nurses and physician rapidly begin to assess the infant for obvious signs of problems. This initial assessment leads to an *Apgar score,* a rating of the infant's basic appearance by one minute of life. In arriving at the Apgar, a score of 0, 1, or 2 is assigned for each of the following five areas: heart rate, respiration, muscle tone, reflex irritability (such as coughing or sneezing), and color. The maximum score is 10 (2 points for each of the five areas assessed). An infant who is not breathing well, is blue or pale, does not cry, or is limp will receive a very low Apgar score and immediate steps will be taken to improve the baby's condition. This rapid assessment is repeated at five minutes after birth, leading to two Apgar scores. The second is expected to be higher than the first.

I typically ask parents the infant's Apgar ratings. It is helpful to know these scores; however, they are less important than an awareness of the baby's condition at the time of birth and shortly thereafter. If, for example, the infant was handed to the mother shortly after birth and the cutting of the umbilical cord, it is likely that there were no significant concerns. On the other hand, an infant who showed persistent signs of oxygen deprivation, slow heart rate, or poor muscle tone was likely whisked away to the nursery for more intensive medical care. This information is more telling than the Apgar scores alone and may be more helpful in determining high-risk factors for APD.

In general, the poorer the infant's health after birth, the more at risk he may be for difficulties later in life. Although such conditions as short-term fetal distress and temporary lack of oxygen are not considered high-risk factors for permanent hearing loss, we do not know whether these factors can disrupt the delicate neurological balance required for precise auditory processing. Therefore, it is important to take into account any health-related difficulties that occurred during the pregnancy, birth, or early life of the child.

All of this leads us to the final key factor in determining whether an infant or very young child may be at risk for an auditory processing problem.

Development of the Child Regardless of the absence of high-risk factors or the outcome of hearing screening measures, infants and young children should be monitored carefully for normal development. Hearing testing should be the first step in determining why a child is not developing speech and language as he should, but the finding of normal hearing acuity does not eliminate the need for further evaluation of speech, language, auditory processing, and other development as soon as possible after such concerns arise. If a problem does exist, intervention should begin at the earliest possible age. That so many of the children we see with APD have virtually no high-risk factors emphasizes the need for careful monitoring of developmental milestones by parents, pediatricians or general practitioners, day-care providers, and others involved in the life of every child. Therefore, it is important that parents and others have an awareness of normal development.

Following are the typical stages of speech and language development in children from birth through age three. This information is intended to be a general guide only and is not to be used for diagnostic purposes. Some children develop all of these skills at earlier ages, and some may not develop a few skills until later. Deviations from the following milestones occur frequently in children who do not have a disorder of speech, language, or hearing, or in children who were premature at birth. However, significant delays may raise a suspicion of some type of speech/language or auditory processing problem and may require follow-up. (Information compiled from the American Speech-Language-Hearing Association consumer information Web site, www.asha.org; Mary Brooks and Deedra Engmann-Hartung's speech and language development brochures, Pro-Ed of Austin, Texas, (512) 451-3246; and *What to Expect the First Year* and *What to Expect the Toddler Years* by Arlene Eisenberg, Heidi E. Murkoff, and Sandee E. Hathaway, Workman Publishing.)

TYPICAL STAGES OF SPEECH AND LANGUAGE DEVELOPMENT FROM BIRTH THROUGH AGE THREE

At birth, the child

- Startles to loud or unexpected sounds

- Cries when uncomfortable, hungry, or wet

- May calm to a familiar, comforting voice

- May cease behavior when he hears a new sound

At six months, the child

- Makes many different sounds, including laughing, gurgling, and cooing

- Reacts to tone of voice, especially if loud or angry

- Turns (or localizes) in the direction of new sounds

- Enjoys toys that make noise, such as rattles or squeakers, musical toys, and being sung to

- Babbles to get attention, using consonants such as *p, b,* and *m*

- Smiles when he is spoken to

- Indicates that he wants something through sound or gesture

At eight months, the child

- Responds to his or her name

- Says at least four or more different, distinct sounds

- Uses syllables such as *da, ba, ka*

- Listens to his or her own voice and others' voices

- Tries to imitate some sounds

- Responds to *no*

- Enjoys participating in games such as peekaboo and pat-a-cake

At ten months, the child

- *May* say *mama* or *dada,* but does not necessarily apply the correct label to the person

- Shouts, squeals, or uses some other vocal, noncrying sound to attract attention

- Uses connected syllables that sound like real speech in their general intonation and consonant-vowel makeup, including both long and short groups of sounds

- Repeats certain syllables or sequences of sounds over and over

At one year, the child

- Recognizes his name and turns to look when his name is called

- Says *mama* and *dada* and may have two or three additional words in his vocabulary

- Imitates familiar words and animal sounds

- Understands simple instructions (such as "Give me . . ." or "Come here")

- Waves (and understands) *bye-bye*

- Makes appropriate eye contact and shows affection for familiar people

- Responds to sounds such as the doorbell ringing or the dog barking

- Understands that words are symbols for objects (e.g., shows that the word *dog* refers to the furry, funny-looking beast beneath his high chair by pointing; points to pictures in a book when named)

- Understands (but does not always agree with) the word *no*

At eighteen months, the child

- Uses at least five to ten words, including names of people and familiar things

- Uses some words to express wants or needs (e.g., "More"), but also often points or gestures to the desired object

- Begins to combine two words (e.g., "All gone")

- Points to familiar body parts

- Recognizes pictures of familiar things and people

- Gets a familiar object upon request, even if it is in another room

- Imitates sounds and words more accurately

- Hums or sings simple tunes

- Hears and responds to quiet speech

At two years, the child

- Uses two- to three-word "sentences," including negative sentences such as "No want" and "No go"

- Has approximately two hundred to three hundred words in his vocabulary, uses at least fifty to one hundred words regularly

- Expresses simple desires or needs for familiar things or actions through speaking rather than pointing (e.g., "More cookie," "Want up")

- Refers to self by name rather than *me* or *I*

- Asks *wh* questions (such as "What that?" and "Where kitty?")

- Understands simple questions and commands

- Names familiar pictures

At two and a half years, the child

- Has a four-hundred-word vocabulary and can name familiar objects and pictures

- Says his first name and holds up fingers to show his age

- Says *no,* but may mean *yes*

- Refers to himself as *me* rather than by name

- Answers *where* questions

- Uses short sentences regularly, such as "Me do it"

- Uses past tense and plurals, although not always correctly (e.g., *drawed, foots*)

- Talks to other children and adults

- Can match at least three colors

- Knows big and little

At three years, the child

- Should be intelligible to strangers, even though many articulation errors may persist

- Has a vocabulary of nearly a thousand words (that is, has a word for almost everything) and speaks in three- to four-word sentences

- Names at least one color, can match all primary colors

- Knows concepts such as night and day, boy and girl, big and little, in and on, up and down, go and stop

- Follows two-step requests such as "Get the toy and put it in the box"

- Can sing familiar songs

- Talks a lot (to himself and others)

- Expresses abstract thoughts, ideas, and concepts verbally and can tell a short story to another person

- Asks *what* and *why* questions

- Can hear his name when called from another room

- Can hear the television or radio at the same level as others in the family

Again, it should be emphasized that these are but general guidelines. Children develop at different paces, and these differences can, quite naturally, prompt questions and concerns. Here are some of the most common questions I hear from parents, and their answers.

FREQUENTLY ASKED QUESTIONS

If my child isn't doing all of the things on the checklists, does this mean that she has an APD or speech/language disorder? Not necessarily. Some children are late bloomers, or shy and not as talkative as other children. In addition, children understand far more than they can produce, even at an early age. Therefore, it is important to pay attention to how your child responds to sounds in the environment, how well she seems to understand what is said and how well she follows simple commands or requests. It is also important to remember that infants and young children produce what they hear. Therefore, although many three-year-olds can sing "Twinkle, Twinkle, Little Star," they would not be expected to do so if they haven't been exposed to that song. Nor would they be expected to know the names for things not present in their environment, no matter how familiar such items seem to the rest of us. Finally, remember that, although speech and language delays may arise from an APD, that is not always the case. The most important factor to consider is whether the child is more or less on target for the majority of skills, and whether she is progressing and regularly adding new words to her vocabulary.

What can I do to stimulate my baby's speech and language development? In a word, talk, talk, talk. Infants need to be talked to, sung to, played with, and stimulated from the moment they are born. Stimulation allows the brain to build strong connections, so always respond enthusiastically to an infant's babbling and cooing. Sing songs and recite nursery rhymes, read books aloud even when the child is too young to participate, play games such as peekaboo and pat-a-cake, point out and name familiar objects, actions, and sounds, and expose the child to new situations and environments. In short, make sure that infants and toddlers are active participants in this rich, engaging, complex world from the moment they take their first breath. Parents should talk naturally to their child, discussing what he is doing and what he sees around him. Parents should also take time to listen, and to respond when the child makes sounds or vocalizes. Finally, don't push your child or force him to talk correctly. Speech errors are a normal part of development and should not immediately be corrected; however, *modeling* of the correct production and *expansion* of the sentence may be helpful if done so that the child does not feel as if he has made a mistake. Modeling involves actually demonstrating the correct way the word or sentence should be produced without drawing attention to the error. Expansion refers to adding on and enriching the child's utterance to expand his exposure to related concepts and words. For example, if the child says, "Me drawed it," referring to a scribble on a paper, the parent can say, "Oh, you drew [modeling] a beautiful, blue picture for me [expansion]." Allow your child to feel that talking and interacting is an enjoyable experience. Make talking fun.

If I think that my child is not talking as much as she should, when should I seek help? Parents know their children better than anyone else, so they are the best people to look for signs that their child may not be progressing as should be expected. Heed your instincts. Follow up on your concerns, either by requesting a referral for assessment services or by seeking out such services independently. If a problem exists, intervention can begin as soon as it is identified.

Whom should I turn to if I do have a concern about my child's hearing or language? Speech and language delays or disorders can arise from many factors, one of which is APD. However, the only way to determine the nature of a child's difficulties is to obtain the appropriate diagnostic services, which requires engaging the child's primary-care physician and the services of the speech-language pathologist and audiologist, as well as any other professionals needed to assess the child's development. The speech-language pathologist is uniquely qualified to address disorders of speech or language. The audiologist is uniquely qualified to address disorders of hearing. Although the primary-care physician or other professional may provide insight and information regarding his or her impressions of the child's development in these areas, only the speech-language pathologist and audiologist can actually diagnose and treat disorders of speech, language, and hearing.

Under the Individuals with Disabilities Education Act (IDEA), which was reauthorized by Congress and signed into law in 1997, states are required to develop programs that provide appropriate early-intervention services to all infants and toddlers with disabilities and their families. The first step in this process is *child find,* or the identification of children with disabilities. These statewide systems are designed to assess infants and toddlers from birth to age three who are suspected of developmental delays. Assessment and intervention services should be accessible to all individuals regardless of socioeconomic status or geographic location. For more information regarding accessing services in the areas of speech, language, and hearing in your area, you may speak to your primary-care physician or contact your state's department of education, local university speech and hearing clinic, or the American Speech-Language-Hearing Association at 1-800-638-8255 (Web site: www.asha.org).

APD DIAGNOSIS IN THE INFANT OR TODDLER

Most behavioral tests for APD cannot be administered until the child is at least seven. Therefore, the child's early speech and language development, along with how he responds to sound in his environment, may represent virtually all of the information we have to determine if an APD may be present in a very young child. A multidisciplinary team is necessary to determine the nature of a child's speech and language difficulties, hearing status, and development in other areas involving sensory and motor skills. This team, which may include audiologists, speech-language pathologists, physicians, early-childhood specialists, psychologists, occupational and physical therapists, and anyone else who works with very young children, will be critical in attempting to understand why a toddler or very young child may be having difficulty communicating. Information from a variety of professionals, when viewed as a whole, may help us determine whether a young child's problems suggest an auditory processing deficit or other causes.

APD frequently does not become apparent until a child enters preschool or even elementary school. In some cases, APD does not fully manifest itself until language demands become much more difficult, such as in high school or even college. Even if the APD is identified early in life, the ways in which it impacts the child's ability to learn and communicate will be different depending on his or her age and school setting.

BUILDING BLOCKS: APD AND THE PRESCHOOL CHILD

The transition from "toddler" to "preschool-aged child" makes us take a step back and look with new eyes at this small person. Just yesterday, he was a baby, and now, seemingly overnight, he has become a "big kid." Suddenly, entirely new expectations are placed on the child. There are behaviors and skills that he is expected to learn. And there are rules: rules for snack time, for sharing, for nap time, for general behavior. Although children might have had some exposure to these conditions during their toddler years (especially if they were in day care), now the rules become stricter, the schedules more circumscribed, the activities more organized. Less time is spent in free play, and more attention is given to learning specific, pre-academic skills. Children learn to match and name primary colors. They learn not only to sing the alphabet, but also to say each letter and to associate each with its corresponding written symbol. They learn to recognize their own name in writing, to color with a crayon, and to write some letters. A number of children now learn basic computer skills in preschool, something that was inconceivable just a few short years ago. They can manipulate the mouse, click on icons, and play computer or video games better than many of their parents! Today, many children enter full-day kindergarten programs already reading at a primer level or even higher. In short, much more is expected of the preschool-aged child today than in past generations.

In one sense, this emphasis on performance at such an early age makes it easier for us to identify warning signs of possible learning or auditory processing problems in younger children. On the other hand, this current emphasis on academics at such a young age may place undue stress on some children, especially those who have some type of language or auditory disorder.

All of us must realize that, although some children are early starters in pre-academic skills, even reading and writing rather fluently during preschool, children develop at their own pace. Never forget that each child is an individual, with individual strengths and weaknesses. Some children may be good at socializing and creative play, but have no interest in pre-reading or writing activities or rule-oriented games. Others may thrive on art or music, but truly dislike playing tag or getting dirty in the sandbox.

The emphasis placed on early pre-academic skill development in many preschool settings sometimes fails to acknowledge that children from three to five years old are as different from one another as oranges and pomegranates. Parents should try not to compare their own children's performance against that of the "high achievers" in the preschool class. They should look at their child's strengths and weaknesses across many areas, including play skills, social communication, and other nonacademic abilities and determine whether steady progress is being made, whether new concepts are being developed and new skills learned, and whether the child is on target for expected speech, language, and related developmental milestones.

When my oldest child was about three years old, we were at a large holiday gathering and she was playing with a set of dominoes with another child who was about the same age. As the adults watched, my daughter stacked the dominoes and arranged them in various patterns, declaring that she was making a house, a dog, a car. The other child, a little boy who was very rule-oriented, told her that this was not how dominoes was played and tried to teach her the correct way. My daughter, however, had no interest in matching numbers of dots. Instead, she continued to arrange the small rectangles in patterns that made sense to her, but this infuriated the little boy because it violated his idea of appropriate organization.

An argument ensued, and the dominoes were taken away and the children provided with crayons and paper instead. While the little boy began to carefully write the letters of his name, my daughter scribbled all over her paper with a gray crayon, then drew bold black slashes through the gray background. When asked what she was drawing, she replied, "I'm drawing thunder." At that, the little boy pointed out, rather imperiously, "You can't draw thunder 'cause you can't see it." He then turned his attention back to meticulously writing his name and other simple words.

I was rather amused by this little exchange, but my amusement quickly faded when one of the adults in our group said to the little boy, within full range of my daughter's hearing, "It's okay, honey. Let it go. *She's just not as smart as you are.*"

Several other adults in the room nodded and murmured in agreement.

Of course, this angered me. And when I saw the look of hurt confusion that came over my daughter's face, my anger rapidly became fury. I retorted, childishly perhaps—but justifiably—"And *he's* not as *creative* as *she* is." I then took my daughter into the kitchen for cookies and milk. This incident still infuriates me, and holiday gatherings have never been quite the same since.

The little boy *was* far more advanced in the traditional learning-based, pre-academic skills than my daughter was. But, I preferred— indeed, was thrilled—that my child at age three was able to see infinite patterns in dominoes and visualize or draw things that could only be heard. In today's world, however, greater emphasis is placed on skills such as reading and spelling than on the more creative abilities that show cognitive processes related to abstract thought and mental flexibility. Although laypeople consider the early ability to read and write to be an index of how "smart" a child is, research has shown that overall cognitive ability is actually more related to the types of imaginative thought my daughter was showing at age three. Indeed, today my daughter is talented both academically and in music, art, and creative writing.

The lesson to be learned here is that, although we may be tempted to equate the early development of pre-academic skills with high cognitive ability or learning capacity in the preschool child, it is important to recognize that young children show what they know in very different ways. Their likes and dislikes will affect the types of activities at which they excel. Therefore, what is most important is that the child is healthy, happy, and developing at a pace that is typical of other children the same age. So, let's not focus just yet on what the child *may* be able to do in preschool. Let us, instead, focus on what he *should* be able to do. Here is a summary of speech, language, and related abilities that are typical of preschool-aged children. Once again, this information is intended as a general guide only. A parent or caregiver who has any concerns that a child is not developing as expected should seek assistance as soon as the concern arises.

NORMAL SPEECH AND LANGUAGE DEVELOPMENT IN PRESCHOOL-AGED CHILDREN

At four years, the child

- Has a vocabulary of fifteen hundred words
- Uses four-to-five-word sentences
- Begins to use more complex sentences
- Uses plurals, contractions, and past tense
- Asks many questions, including "Why?"
- Understands simple *who, what,* and *where* questions
- Can follow commands and directions, even if the target object is not present
- Can identify some basic shapes (e.g., circle, square)
- Can identify primary colors
- Can talk about concepts in the abstract and imaginary conditions (e.g., "I hope Santa brings me a scooter")
- Begins to copy patterns on a page (e.g., lines, circles)
- Pays attention to a short story and may be able to answer questions about it
- Hears and understands most of what is said at home and in school

- Relates incidents that happened in school or at home (e.g., "Jimmy hit me")

At five years, the child

- Has a vocabulary of two thousand words

- Uses five-to-six-word sentences

- Produces most speech sounds correctly (except for the later-developing ones)

- Uses all types of sentences, including complex ones that describe cause and effect or temporal relations (e.g., "I'll get in trouble if I hit Jimmy" or "I can have a cookie after I eat my lunch") and sentences that incorporate past, present, and future tense

- Can count to ten (including counting number of objects)

- Can tell what objects are used for and made of and knows spatial relations (e.g., on top of, behind, far, near)

- Knows opposite concepts (hard/soft, long/short, same/different)

- Asks questions for the purpose of gaining new information

- Knows right and left on himself, but not necessarily on others

- Can express feelings, dreams, wishes, and other abstract thoughts

- Can copy basic capital letters when shown a model, *may* be able to write name, can draw rudimentary pictures

- Again, hears and understands most of what is said at home and in school

Although some children may be able to spell or read some by age five, those skills are not the norm at this stage. Children should, however, understand the concepts that books have words and that words are made up of letters. They may also begin to demonstrate the knowledge that certain letters correspond to certain sounds. For example, most five-year-old children are less likely to be satisfied with merely looking at the pictures in a favorite book, but will instead bring it to a parent or an older sibling with the request "Will you read it to me?" They may even make up stories corresponding to the pictures and relate them aloud as they turn the pages. Most five-year-olds can recognize their own name in writing. Some can even write it. Although most of them can sing the alphabet song, they are not always able to *say* the alphabet letter by letter.

When looking for warning signs that an APD may be present in a preschool child, we should first look at whether the child is exhibiting normal speech and language milestones. Just as with the infant and the toddler, the child's speech and language development provides us with the best information on how the preschool child may be hearing, processing, and using speech. Once again, however, we should note that language or articulation difficulties do not necessarily mean that an APD is present; only careful multidisciplinary assessment can determine the nature of the difficulties a child may be having. We should also verify that the child is adding new vocabulary regularly and progressing steadily in the complexity of sentences that he can both produce and understand.

It is worth mentioning the relationship between childhood illness and hearing acuity in the preschool child. Children may be exposed to new illnesses for the first time in preschool, especially if they have not been around many children previously. Viruses, colds, and ear infections are common in preschool children. In fact, 50 percent of children will have had at least one ear infection before they are a year old, and 35 percent will have repeated infections between the first and third years. Ear infections are one of the most common conditions in preschool- and school-aged children, second only to the common cold.

As you probably know from experience, you don't hear well when your ears are plugged up. Similarly, an ear infection can affect a child's hearing acuity, and the child may miss important information in school or at home. This is true even if the child's hearing has been tested previously and found to be completely normal. Therefore, it is important for parents and caregivers to keep an eye out for any signs that a child may be having difficulty hearing, such as saying "Huh?" or "What?" or requesting that the television be tuned louder.

Ear infections occur more frequently in very young children because the Eustachian tube, which runs between the middle ear and the back of the throat, is narrower and more horizontally positioned in children. This tube can become blocked more easily by inflammation associated with colds, tonsillitis, and other upper-respiratory conditions, which makes children more susceptible to ear infections.

It is often possible to tell when a small child has an ear infection. The child may have a fever, complain of pain, or if too young to verbalize, may pull at his ears and cry. He may also exhibit other obvious signs of illness such as crankiness, lethargy, or lack of appetite. However, some ear infections are "silent" and may thus go undetected. Ear infections are associated with a buildup of fluid behind the eardrum, and if this fluid contains bacteria, other signs of infection and general illness will usually accompany the infection. However, if the fluid does not contain bacteria, a decrease in hearing acuity may be the only symptom, and that can easily go unnoticed. If an undetected ear infection persists for long enough, the fluid in the middle ear may become very thick, a condition known as glue-ear, and result in more serious effects on hearing sensitivity.

It is possible even for a physician to miss clear, uninfected fluid in the middle ear by looking into the ear with an otoscope, especially if there is no redness or inflammation of the eardrum, no "fluid line" as often occurs when the middle ear is completely full of fluid, and no air bubbles in the fluid. Therefore, chronic ear infections with no associated symptoms may not be detected during routine visits to the pediatrician. Furthermore, although annual hearing screening is conducted at most preschools and many day-care centers, a child may not have any ear problems at the time of the screening and then develop an ear infection the very next day, particularly during the winter months. That a child has passed a hearing screening does not mean that a hearing problem may not occur thereafter.

Children learn an incredible amount in a relatively short time in these formative years. Therefore, any condition that can affect their ability to hear clearly can, likewise, affect their speech, language, and auditory processing abilities. Chronic or persistent ear infections have been linked to speech and language delays and auditory processing deficits in some children. Children who have "silent" ear infections appear to be most at risk because their mild hearing losses may be present for longer periods before they are detected. That's why one of the JCIH risk factors for hearing loss is recurrent or persistent ear infections with fluid for at least three months.

Parents and caregivers should be vigilant in looking for signs that a child may have a middle ear problem that can affect hearing. Some of these symptoms include

- Inattentiveness

- Wanting the television or radio louder than usual

- Pulling or scratching at the ears

- Difficulty following directions or understanding what is being said that is not typical for the child, including saying "Huh?" or "What?"

- Unexplained irritability

- Making comments about how the ears feel strange (the first tip-off that my youngest son had an ear infection recently was his saying, "My ears are beeping." I still don't know what he meant by that, but sure enough, he had an ear infection with fluid but without fever or pain)

If you suspect that persistent ear infections are causing a speech, language, or auditory processing problem in a child, you should take a multidisciplinary approach involving a physician, a speech-language pathologist, and an audiologist. The physician will deal with the medical treatment of the infection(s), possibly even suggesting surgery to put tubes in the eardrums that will allow the fluid to drain. This procedure has a high success rate and results in rapid improvement in hearing, particularly in those children for whom traditional treatment with antibiotics or other approaches have been unsuccessful for three months or so. The speech-language pathologist will address the specific speech and language difficulties or delays the child may be having. Finally, the audiologist will assess hearing acuity, middle ear function, and may address concerns related to auditory processing by analyzing how the child responds to auditory stimuli during the test session and in the environment.

In summary, key red flags that an auditory processing problem might be present in a preschool-aged child are similar to those for the infant and the toddler. That is, does the child demonstrate achievement of speech and language milestones at appropriate ages? Does the child seem to respond to auditory stimuli appropriately? Can he follow directions? Does he ask for repetitions or say "Huh?" or "What?" a lot? We should also continue to address the issue of hearing acuity, especially the transient or fluctuating hearing loss that may accompany chronic ear infections in some youngsters. Even if the child has no history of ear infections or hearing loss, does the child, nevertheless, act as though he isn't hearing as well or as clearly as he should?

WARNING SIGNS OF APD IN PRESCHOOL CHILDREN

Below is an easy-to-follow checklist of warning signs that may signal an APD. I have based this short list on the most common signs or symptoms shown by preschool children with APD; however, these signs or symptoms do *not* necessarily mean that an APD *is* present, only that it *may* be. If you have any concern about your child's auditory processing or related abilities, seek appropriate follow-up services at once. Bear in mind that these behaviors can occur for any number of reasons and that APD cannot be diagnosed from a checklist, no matter how well the child seems to "fit" the behaviors described. Nevertheless, preschool-aged children with APD *may*

- Demonstrate delayed speech and language abilities, or articulation errors that are not consistent with age or that suggest acoustic confusions (such as substituting *d* for *g*)

- Have difficulty following directions at school or at home that other children of the same age are able to follow easily (e.g., "Put your crayons away and line up for play time")

- Have an easier time following daily routines (once they are learned), such as putting a coat in a cubby upon arriving at school or getting a blanket from the closet for quiet time, than following new, verbally presented information or instructions

- Ask for repetitions frequently, such as "Huh?" or "What?" Of course, "Huh?" can mean a lot of things when coming from a small child, including, "I didn't hear you," "I didn't understand you," "I already forgot what you said," "I really don't want to do that," or even "I wasn't paying attention because the cartoon on TV is way more interesting than you are." It may be difficult, if not impossible, to distinguish among these causes without paying close attention to the types of situations during which the child asks for repetitions

- Demonstrate signs of frustration or confusion, running the gamut from refusing to participate to staring back with a completely blank face, when confronted with new instructions or activities

- Perform better when a visual example of the expected activity or behavior is provided, that is, when *shown* rather than *told* what to do

- Have relatively greater difficulty understanding instructions or orally presented stories when the environment is noisy

- Fail to keep up with the increasing complexity of verbally presented information in school as kindergarten approaches, even if he was able to follow simpler directions at a younger age

- Have difficulty learning nursery rhymes or simple songs, including singing the ABC's

- Show a complete lack of awareness that books have words and words are made up of letters, even after extended exposure to the topic (e.g., demonstrating no interest in having a book read to him or ignoring the text entirely)

- Demonstrate social communication difficulties, such as hurt feelings or frequent misunderstandings, more often than other children (remember, however, that children are sensitive and frequently get into arguments or complain that another child has mistreated them or hurt their feelings)

- Avoid talking with other children or adults

- Be highly distractible, especially in noisy situations

- Have an easier time with "nonverbal" concepts such as color matching and counting

- Fail to exhibit steady progression in production and/or comprehension of more complex language and new vocabulary (e.g., don't begin to use new words for things even after repeated exposures or fail to keep up with their peers in the types and length of words and sentences produced and understood)

- Fail to respond to or show curiosity about new sounds or demonstrate no attention or interest when spoken to

The most common complaint I hear from parents or caregivers of preschoolers with APD, nonspecific as it may seem, is that they just don't seem to "get it," that the connections just don't appear to be happening as expected. Parents tend to know when something is wrong with their child, when she is not progressing at her true level. Only careful assessment by appropriate professionals can determine the underlying nature of the difficulties, however, and diagnoses should never be made based on observation alone. Indeed, unless a clear abnormality is present in auditory electrophysiology or other physiologic measures, diagnosing APD in a preschool child is not possible using our current behavioral tools. However, with meticulous multidisciplinary collaboration, along with behavioral observation, we can make an educated hypothesis that a child may be exhibiting an APD and the nature of the APD, allowing us to begin intervention at a very young age—even before a formal diagnosis can be made.

As a child grows and begins to learn new academic skills in school, we have more information to go on than just the child's speech and language development. We are also able to draw from a larger arsenal of central auditory diagnostic test tools once a child reaches seven or eight years of age.

SHOW-AND-TELL:
APD IN ELEMENTARY SCHOOL

Elementary school is a time for show-and-tell, for playing hopscotch on the playground, and learning how to paint. It is also a time for learning to read, write, spell, and solve math problems. Auditory processing is an integral component of many of these skills. Many subtle forms of APD may not manifest themselves until the demands of the learning or communication environment become sufficiently challenging. That's why an APD may suddenly "appear" during elementary school.

The vast majority of children I see for APD assessment or consultation are of elementary-school age. Sometimes, with careful probing, I uncover earlier hints that an auditory problem was present (for example, the occasional difficulty hearing or understanding, especially in noisy backgrounds). But often the first real symptoms of an APD are not apparent until the child is trying to learn new, more advanced skills that rely on, or are associated with, auditory processing.

By the time a child enters the first grade, she should be producing almost all speech sounds correctly, using adultlike grammar in sentences and conversations, and understanding the meaning of most sentences (unless unfamiliar or advanced vocabulary or concepts are introduced). Other skills expected of a six-year-old child include knowing the days of the week, counting to at least thirty, telling a multipart story or predicting the next sequence of events in an unfinished story, knowing when his or her birthday is, and understanding concepts such as today, yesterday, and tomorrow. Children of this age are like little adults—we can talk to them using adultlike grammar and they can respond in kind. The nature of their thoughts and communications will, of course, reveal the child inside. Nevertheless, the *form* of their communication should be similar to that of adults. Children of this age also ask many, many questions and are usually truly interested in the answers, particularly if they illuminate how something works, why something is the way it is, or what a new object or word represents. Thus, most children enter school filled with curiosity.

Sadly, what begins as an exciting adventure into new territory can, for some children, quickly turn into a terrifying roller-coaster ride. What appears to come so easily to others may seem difficult, even incomprehensible, to the child with a learning difficulty. The first time a child with a learning difficulty doesn't understand, can't do it, offers a wrong answer or an off-topic remark to a discussion, or just doesn't *get it*, he is embarrassed. If the struggle continues, the child may be called names on the playground—*stupid, dummy, retard*—and begin to withdraw, to separate himself from the others, or to act out in class so that he can gain a type of attention not focused on his academic difficulties. And all the while he will be aware that this is not how it is supposed to be, that despite his best efforts he has let down his parents, his teacher, and even himself.

Elementary-school-aged children with APD can present many different pictures to the world. There are generally accepted key indicators of possible APD in children of this age; however, virtually no child with APD exhibits all of these signs and some exhibit few, if any. In addition, because some of these key indicators are so common in children with other types of disorders involving everything from attention-deficit to behavioral-conduct disorders, lists of symptoms should never be used for diagnostic purposes, but only to raise suspicion that an APD might be present.

Elementary-school children with APD *may*

- Behave as if a hearing loss is present, despite normal hearing acuity, especially in noisy environments

- Demonstrate greater difficulty with verbal than nonverbal tasks, with verbal IQ lower than performance IQ

- Demonstrate significant scatter, or fluctuation in ability levels, across tests of speech, language, or cognitive processes, with weaknesses in those areas considered to be more auditory in nature

- Exhibit a delay in the content, use, or form of language

- Exhibit articulation errors that persist longer than they should

- Be distractible

- Refuse to participate in classroom discussions or, conversely, offer inappropriate or off-topic contributions

- Exhibit difficulty following multistep directions

- Demonstrate poor reading or spelling skills

- Have a history of chronic ear infections, head trauma, or other ear- or brain-related condition

- Exhibit poor music or singing skills

- Require a high degree of external organization in the classroom to begin and complete required tasks

- Exhibit poor social communication skills or difficulty making and keeping friends

- Rely heavily on memorization when learning new information or skills

- Demonstrate inappropriate behavior, including withdrawal, acting out, tantruming, clowning, or playing instead of completing the task at hand

- Express frustration with certain tasks, such as saying "I can't do this" or "I don't understand"

- Demonstrate poor problem-solving skills

- Perform better when auditory information is augmented with visual or tactile cues

Most children exhibit some of these behaviors at some time. Getting frustrated, clowning around in class, and distractibility are common characteristics of elementary-school kids. For the child with an APD, however, these behaviors are both more consistent and more

frequent *as compared with other children of the same age*. Even more important, children with APD rarely exhibit *all* of these behaviors. Indeed,
when I see a child who fits every single item on this list, I begin to suspect other causes either in addition to, or instead of, APD. The behaviors of children with APD tend to follow specific patterns, as will be
seen below, with some types of behaviors being more likely to occur
together in an individual child than others.

KEY INDICATORS OF APD IN THE ELEMENTARY-SCHOOL CHILD

**Behaving as if a hearing loss is present, despite normal hearing acuity,
especially in noisy environments.** This is considered *the* classic hallmark of APD. The most common complaint by far that we hear from
children and adults with APD is difficulty hearing in backgrounds of
noise, a complaint that is also common to people with hearing loss. A
hearing loss causes distortions in what is heard, with some speech
sounds being heard more clearly than others. Moreover, when a person has a hearing loss, much of the incoming message may simply not
be heard at all. APD is somewhat like a hearing loss that occurs not in
the ear, but in the auditory pathways or the brain. The child with an
APD, like the child with a hearing loss, may hear a distorted or incomplete message. Background noise causes even more distortion and cov-
ers up, or masks, more of the message. As a result, the child with an
APD who is trying to listen to a speaker in a noisy room has little to
go on when trying to fill in the missing pieces and achieve auditory
closure.

And yet not all children with APD exhibit this symptom, which by
itself does not provide much insight into what type of APD may be
present. This is because almost any problem in listening or processing
auditory information will be far more pronounced when the environment is so noisy that even normal listeners have some difficulty hearing. Also, difficulty hearing in noise may be due to many factors other

than APD. For example, the child with attention-deficit/hyperactivity disorder (AD/HD) most certainly will have greater difficulty listening in noisy or distracting situations and may appear at times as if he has a hearing loss because he misses much of what is said.

If a child is exhibiting symptoms that suggest he has a hearing loss, the first step should be to make sure that he *doesn't* have a hearing loss. The child may be experiencing a hearing loss due to an ear infection or for a host of other reasons. Therefore, a complete hearing evaluation is critical when difficulties with listening or hearing are suspected. Finally, it is important to note that not all individuals with APD have normal hearing acuity. APD can coexist with hearing loss and render activities such as listening in noise even more difficult than they would have been if the hearing loss had occurred alone. Therefore, we should not assume that an APD is present merely because the child acts as though he has a hearing loss or exhibits difficulty hearing in noise. Only appropriate diagnostic follow-up can shed light on the reasons underlying these types of listening problems.

Behaviors consistent with hearing loss include asking frequently for repetitions, including saying "Huh?" or "What?" and responding to questions or instructions incorrectly. However, these behaviors may also occur if the child just didn't happen to hear what was said, didn't understand what was said, or forgot what was said soon after hearing it. Sometimes children can differentiate between these underlying meanings of "Huh?" with careful probing and guidance. For example, a child may say, "I couldn't hear what you said." Alternatively, he may say, "I heard you, but I don't know what you mean." Finally, he may say, "I knew what I was supposed to do, but I started playing with the cat and I forgot." Encouraging the child to self-analyze and make statements such as these can help us understand what a child really means by "Huh?" or "What?"

Demonstrating greater difficulty with verbal than nonverbal tasks, with verbal IQ lower than performance IQ. Most often, a child with an APD will have difficulty with subjects such as reading and written language, social studies, and science. Laboratory exercises or hands-on demonstrations are usually the exception as these activities may provide sufficient tactile and visual cues to compensate for the auditory deficit. The student with an APD will likely be compromised in his ability to listen to, comprehend, and answer questions about stories or topics presented in class. A child with an APD usually performs better in math, art, and music.

These symptoms are most characteristic of children with APD involving the left hemisphere of the brain. This is because, for most people, the left hemisphere is dominant for language. In contrast, the right hemisphere is typically dominant for activities that are not as reliant on language. Therefore, an APD that involves the right hemisphere may lead to a completely opposite pattern of difficulties. Children with right-hemisphere-based APD may have problems with mathematics calculation, music, and art. In fact, for these children, performance in more verbal-based subjects may be far better than in nonverbal-based subjects. When standardized psychoeducational or cognitive testing is carried out, children with right-hemisphere-based APD may exhibit higher verbal IQ scores than nonverbal IQ scores. This is because nonverbal IQ scales usually involve such activities as copying patterns with blocks, visual perception tasks, completing puzzles, and creating whole objects from many parts—all activities that rely more on the right side of the brain than the left.

Finally, when the two hemispheres of the brain are not working together—a condition known as inefficient interhemispheric integration—a different pattern of academic difficulties may emerge. A child with an APD resulting from inefficient interhemispheric integration may exhibit difficulty with any subject that requires both halves of the brain to work together cooperatively, whether verbal or nonverbal. Thus, these children may exhibit difficulties in coordinating both hands or feet together; problems during physical education class; art and music difficulties; and other difficulties that would not typically be considered indicative of an APD. On the other hand, they may do very well with less complex tasks that rely primarily on one hemisphere of the brain, such as using one foot or hand at a time, recognizing visual patterns, or reciting poetry. For these reasons, we must be very careful of overgeneralizing the common symptom of "verbal abilities poorer than nonverbal abilities" when attempting to determine whether a child may have an APD. Although considered one of the more classic hallmarks of APD, this symptom is not always present, and indeed, some children with APD exhibit the completely opposite pattern. It all depends on the underlying nature of the APD.

Demonstrating an overall pattern of weakness in areas considered more auditory in nature. When a learning disorder or other type of disability is suspected in a child, multidisciplinary testing is usually carried out. Such testing typically involves a speech-language pathologist, audiologist, psychologist, occupational or physical therapist, social worker, and perhaps others. If the results of all tests show the same or similar levels of delay or difficulty, regardless of the type of task involved (e.g., visual, auditory, motor, tactile), test results are said to be *commensurate* with one another. For example, a child with significant delays in all areas, including both nonverbal and verbal IQ, expressive and receptive language skills, motor and self-help skills, academic achievement (regardless of subject), and associated abilities clearly does not have a processing problem in one sensory skill area, such as APD. This child exhibits symptoms of an overall cognitive delay or disorder. As a result, he will probably be diagnosed with mental retardation or a similar condition instead of a specific processing disorder or learning disability.

On the other hand, if significant discrepancies exist among abilities, with some areas in deficient ranges and other areas within the average range or even higher, we consider this a finding of *scatter*. For example, a child may do well in mathematics, but poorly in reading and writing. Nonverbal IQ may be much higher than verbal IQ. This child is very different from one who exhibits evenly developed skills or difficulties across all areas.

An analysis of the areas of strengths and weaknesses can provide some illumination into the underlying nature of the difficulties the child is having. Typically, children with APD demonstrate scatter in subtests of cognitive testing or across multidisciplinary assessments that, based on the tasks in each subtest or assessment tool, require auditory-based or verbal skills to complete. For example, solving verbally presented math problems requires arithmetic ability but also the ability to hear and understand the problem in the first place. But, as just discussed, we must be aware that many types of APD co-occur with difficulties in areas not traditionally considered auditory-verbal in nature, especially APDs resulting from dysfunction in the right hemisphere or interhemispheric pathways of the brain.

Exhibiting a delay in the content, use, or form of language. APD can lead to a variety of language-related difficulties or delays. Children with APD may have difficulty with *syntax,* or the way in which words are put together to form sentences. They may struggle with connecting words or sentences with their meanings, or *semantics.* Finally, they may exhibit poor use of language, or *pragmatics,* leading to social communication difficulties. These problems can manifest themselves in both understanding (receptive) and producing (expressive) language and can also affect written language abilities. A speech-language pathologist can evaluate a child's language abilities in both domains.

It is important to dissociate those language functions that rely relatively more heavily on the left hemisphere from those that rely on the right hemisphere of the brain in most people. Typically, children (and adults) with left-hemisphere-based APD tend to show difficulties in syntax, semantics, and vocabulary skills. On the other hand, children with right-hemisphere-based APD typically show difficulties in pragmatics, or the way language is *used* in various contexts. For these children, the actual form the language takes and the vocabulary or meaning of the words may be appropriate; however, social communication is affected, including the comprehension and expression of subtle, prosodic elements of speech. In addition, children with right-hemisphere-based APD often have difficulty grasping the main idea of a story or message, likely due to difficulty separating those elements that are stressed during delivery of the message from the unstressed, and therefore less important, elements.

Finally, children with dysfunction in the interhemispheric pathways may have difficulty with general language comprehension and production because of problems linking social-communication and tone-of-voice cues with semantics and syntax, something that is necessary to understand the whole message of any communication. For example, if a person sarcastically says, "Wow, *that's* a great outfit!" most listeners will understand that she really means that the outfit is hideous. A child with interhemispheric integration difficulties may be confused at this intentional discrepancy between tone-of-voice and language content and may miss the meaning of the statement altogether.

Exhibiting articulation errors that persist longer than they should. Some articulation errors are part of normal development. For example, substituting *th* for *s* (commonly termed lisping) is common in young children and is considered a developmental error. On the other hand, consistently substituting speech sounds that are acoustically similar, such as *d* and *g*, long past the age at which these errors would be considered normal may herald the presence of an APD. When we consider the articulation errors of an elementary-school child, we are concerned primarily with errors indicating possible acoustic confusions rather than those arising from developmental issues. For example, the child who substitutes *th* for *s* is of far less concern from an auditory processing perspective than the child who deletes final, unstressed consonants, substitutes similar sounding speech sounds (for example, *d* for *g*), or who exhibits other articulation errors that have no apparent oral-motor or motor planning cause. These articulation errors become of even more concern if similar substitutions or confusions occur in reading or spelling, as they lead us to wonder if the child actually *hears* the difference between the speech sounds. My experience is that articulation errors such as these typically accompany left-hemisphere-based APD and are rarely seen with right-hemisphere-based APD. This makes sense from a neurophysiologic standpoint, as speech-sound representation is primarily a function of the primary (usually left) auditory cortex.

Distractibility. Distractibility may be a hallmark of APD, but it is also a hallmark of many other disorders, the most notable being AD/HD. With AD/HD, a child may be distractible because her mind is elsewhere or because an interesting new thought or event has occurred and the child has diverted her attention from the task at hand to follow the new path. However, distractibility associated with APD usually arises from the way in which noise or competing speech interferes with the ability to understand what is being said. For example, the child with an APD may be unable to listen to one speaker when many others are talking at the same time, even if her thoughts and attention are fully on the conversation at hand. Furthermore, some children with APD may "tune out" once they lose the thread of what is being discussed and turn their attention to something else, such as the paper airplane in their desk or the gerbil in the cage against the window. The greater a child's comprehension difficulties, or the noisier the room, the more likely she is to do this. It is difficult to delineate between the distractible behaviors arising from AD/HD and those associated with APD. To make matters worse, the two disorders frequently co-occur. That's why, in chapter 5, we will discuss the issue of differentially diagnosing AD/HD and APD. This is important because the management and treatment of the two disorders are very different. Remember, too, that all children can be distractible some of the time. Distractibility in an elementary-school child may not indicate any type of disorder unless it occurs frequently and interferes with the child's ability to learn or to understand what is being said.

Refusing to participate in classroom discussions or, conversely, offering inappropriate or off-topic contributions. Most young children love to talk. They want to be included, to be a part of the action, to be one of the gang. To do so, however, they must participate in group activities, such as classroom discussions and social conversations. Watch a young child with an APD during a classroom discussion and you can see his eagerness to contribute to the conversation. He'll wave his hand just like all the other children, hoping the teacher will turn her attention to him and call his name. But if he does not fully understand what the discussion is about, what he says will probably be off-topic.

I once observed a second-grade boy with an APD during a classroom presentation regarding fire safety and what to do if a fire breaks out in your home. At the end of the presentation, the visiting firefighter asked a series of questions, including whether you should go back to get your pets if the house is burning. The boy waved his hand in the air and, when the firefighter nodded at him, regaled the class with a story of the latest antics of his cat and new puppy. He had the general idea—his contribution did deal with pets, at least—but his comments were not directly related to the question that was asked. Thankfully, his teacher was aware of his APD and redirected the child gently without embarrassing him.

What happens more often in these situations, however, is one of three things: The teacher may admonish the child ("Joey, that's *not* what I asked. Now, pay attention"), and the other children will giggle while the child, duly chastised, falls into silence. Alternatively, the other children in the class may find the child's contribution more interesting than the topic being discussed and offer their own contributions to this new direction ("I have a dog and cat, too, and *my* dog . . ."), whereupon the teacher will admonish and redirect the entire class, often drawing attention to the child who started the prob-

lem. Or, finally, the child's off-topic contribution may be met with silence or subtle, transient laughter, and the initial discussion will pro-
ceed as if the child hadn't spoken at all.

None of these approaches are particularly conducive to encouraging
a child to continue participating in classroom discussions. Which is
why, as time goes on, a child with APD may begin to withdraw from
group interactions and refuse to participate. You can see this child's
eagerness disintegrate over time, the excited expression replaced with
one of trepidation, the waving hand replaced with a tentative, half-
hearted raising of the fingers. Eventually, the face becomes blank and
the hand remains in the lap, the eyes cast down at the floor as if pray-
ing that the teacher will *not* call on him, not draw attention to him and
set him up, once again, for public failure. The child who was once so
excited to be a participant may become fearful of even the simplest,
most nonthreatening group discussions or conversations.

Again, off-topic or inappropriate contributions to discussions may
also be seen in the child with AD/HD. Therefore, these behaviors
may result either from the impulsivity that accompanies AD/HD or
from the lack of comprehension that accompanies APD. Likewise, the
child who separates himself from the group activity at hand, preferring
instead to play with a toy he has pulled from his pocket or to stare out
the window at the falling snow, may do so for any number of reasons.
Perhaps he isn't able to follow the conversation and does not want to
risk public failure, as occurs with APD. Perhaps something else has
caught his attention or his thoughts have taken a different path, as occurs with AD/HD. Distinguishing behaviors that arise from AD/HD
from those that arise from APD can be extremely difficult based on
observation alone. Only careful diagnostics and multidisciplinary collaboration can help disentangle the two.

Difficulty following multistep directions. The child who has difficulty
understanding what is being said (for whatever reason) will also have
difficulty when given directions that involve several steps or are com-

plex. Difficulty following multistep directions is a hallmark of APD. However, as with the other key indicators of APD, this type of difficulty can arise from many factors: Does the child not hear the directions in the first place? Does he hear them but not understand precisely what they mean? Does he both hear and understand, but forget them as soon as they are presented? Does he hear, understand, and remember them, but, somewhere in following through, become sidetracked by something else—a new toy, the sight of leaves blowing in the wind outside the window—and never complete the task as directed? Difficulty following multistep directions or comprehending complex information can arise from auditory disorders, language disorders, attention disorders, cognitive disorders that affect memory, executive function disorders that affect planning, and many other factors. Therefore, at the risk of repeating the same caveat ad nauseam, difficulty following multistep directions should not, by itself, be taken as conclusive evidence of an APD.

Demonstrating poor reading or spelling skills. Poor reading or spelling skills are often the primary complaints leading to a suspicion of an APD in an elementary-school child. However, to illuminate the underlying nature of the possible APD, or even to determine whether the difficulty might be due to an APD at all, we must delineate precisely what type of reading or spelling difficulties the child is having. Does the child have a hard time making the connection between speech sounds and letters of the alphabet and exhibit other phonological awareness difficulties? If so, a left-hemisphere-based APD involving speech-sound processing may be present. Does she exhibit appropriate phonological attack strategies, but have difficulty with automatically recognizing those words that should be within her sight word vocabulary? This might occur with right-hemisphere-based APD involving the ability to put all of the pieces together and recognize the whole pattern. Does she exhibit problems with both sight word and word attack abilities, as might happen if interhemispheric processing is an issue? Or are her symptoms much more visual in nature? Does she transpose or reverse letters in reading or writing, have difficulty with number identification as well, or respond better with visual interventions such as the use of colored filters on the page or underlining to aid visual tracking? If so, the problem may not be auditory at all. Reading and spelling problems are common in children with APD, but not all spelling and reading problems are due to APD, and not all children with APD will have difficulties learning to spell or read.

Having a history of chronic ear infections, head trauma, or other ear- or brain-related conditions. Early health problems can result in dysfunction in sensory systems, including the auditory system. Certainly, a history of illness or trauma that is associated with problems in auditory processing—particularly chronic ear infections at an early age— is a huge red flag that an APD may be present. However, that a child has had illness or injury that *may* lead to an auditory processing deficit does not necessarily mean that it *will* lead to one. Therefore, this information, as with all of the factors on this list, should be viewed in light of additional observational data when attempting to determine whether a child may have an APD that requires further follow-up.

Exhibiting poor music or singing skills. Many children with APD have difficulty with verbal-based subjects. We must not forget, however, that some children with right-hemisphere-based APD have far greater difficulty in areas not considered verbal or linguistic. These children may have a hard time singing on-key and may dislike music or singing. Typically, these children also have difficulties in art and possibly in pragmatic (or social use of) language. Difficulty with the production and reception of prosodic, or tone-of-voice, elements of speech may also be present. They may speak or read flatly or in a monotone and may frequently misunderstand the intent, rather than the content, of others' communications, leading to hurt feelings or overreaction.

Not all of us can sing like Beverly Sills or appreciate the finer elements of a violin concerto, so the presence of poor singing or musical abilities should not, in itself, be taken as evidence of an APD. Moreover, difficulties in interhemispheric function can also lead to specific musical difficulties, especially playing instruments that require bimanual coordination (such as the piano) or linking the symbolic language of written musical notation with the vocal or manual output. Interhemispheric dysfunction can also affect the ability to comprehend the meaning of the lyrics of a song while, at the same time, appreciating the melody of the music.

Requiring a high degree of external organization in the classroom to begin and complete required tasks. Because they often have difficulty comprehending instructions, children with APD may need to be *shown* what to do, step by step, before they can begin and follow through on a task. Others may have difficulty sequencing the required steps even once they are demonstrated. These children may find it helpful to have a written checklist to refer to. On the other hand, difficulty remembering and following through on simple, routine tasks such as taking their assigned place in the line to go to recess or lunch, putting coats and backpacks in the appropriate cubbies or lockers at the beginning of the day, and knowing where crayons or markers are located in their desks should raise a suspicion of some type of higher-order difficulty rather than a purely auditory disorder. Unless the APD coexists with another, higher-order cognitive or attention dysfunction, children with APD typically do quite well with learned, simple, routine tasks such as these once they know and understand what is expected of them.

Exhibiting poor social communication skills or difficulty making and keeping friends. Our ability to interact and develop relationships with those around us is not fully realized until (and unless) we are able to communicate effectively. We have an innate need to share dreams and thoughts, to talk about what is seen or heard, to reach out with words to connect with others. Even in elementary school, this need is apparent—show-and-tell in kindergarten involves not just demonstrating, but *talking* about something of importance to the child.

If a child has any type of communication problem, including APD, the ability to connect with others will be affected. As the child grows, the need to understand more subtle forms of communication, including humor and sarcasm, becomes an intricate part of interacting with others. If the child is unable to pick up on these subtleties, such as occurs with right-hemisphere-based disorders, he may misunderstand, complain of hurt feelings, and strike out at other children with no apparent provocation. A seven-year-old boy with an APD may be able to share in the obvious, visual-pratfall humor of the Three Stooges, but he may not get more subtle jokes and, as a result, feel left out while his peers laugh uproariously. Alternatively, he may himself tell jokes that aren't funny, either not understanding what constitutes humor or having difficulty delivering the punch line with the appropriate inflection. His attempts to be part of the group, to entertain his peers, may be met with blank stares or, worse, laughter that is directed *at* him, rather than *with* him. Furthermore, children with right-hemisphere-based APD may exhibit other deficits in social judgment that just compound the social communication difficulties brought on by the auditory disorder.

Most social communication in elementary school occurs on the playground or in the lunchroom—places that are very noisy. The child with an APD that affects his ability to hear and discriminate speech, especially in noisy backgrounds, may find it difficult to interact socially at the specific times and places during the school day when such interaction is expected and encouraged. Although we tend to think of school, even elementary school, as being primarily a place to learn the three R's, for a young child, elementary school is the first place where she begins to learn the delicate steps in the social dance of life. Difficulty in making or keeping friends, in using words and language to share, in learning and executing those delicate steps, in simply *connecting* with other kids, may be more devastating to the child's self-image and emotional well-being than difficulty in any other arena.

Relying heavily on memorization when learning new information or skills. Many children with APD demonstrate the greatest difficulty with *new*, unfamiliar information presented verbally or in writing. In contrast, once they have reviewed the information and become familiar with it, they may do well. A child with speech-sound-based APD may obtain 100 percent on spelling tests, yet be unable to spell or decode spontaneously during reading or writing samples. In lower grades, spelling lists are frequently given out on Monday and studied throughout the week, then the children are tested on Thursday or Friday. Many of the children with whom I have worked perform splendidly on these Thursday or Friday spelling tests, but not without a great deal of effort spent in memorizing the words on the list during the week. And unlike their non-APD peers, these children often fail to generalize the spelling rules they were supposed to have learned through this exercise to other similarly spelled words or even to the same words presented in a different context.

This overreliance on memorization, which can manifest itself in the ability to regurgitate facts and figures verbatim, can result in the inability to apply the underlying concepts to new situations or information, since the concepts weren't understood in the first place. Because of the need to memorize, many children with APD spend much more time completing homework assignments than their friends, even in very early grades. Unfortunately, because so much of the grading in all levels of school is based on how well the child spits back facts during written exams, a child who is poor at auditory processing but good at memorizing may go undetected because he achieves at a level appropriate for his age or grade on these types of exams.

Demonstrating inappropriate behavior, including withdrawal, acting out, tantruming, clowning, or playing instead of completing the task at hand. We have talked about this issue to some degree previously, but it bears repeating. A child who is having difficulty hearing or comprehending what is being discussed may respond to his difficulties in a variety of ways. Some children simply tune out and withdraw when they are having difficulty. Others may attempt to gain attention or be part of the group by becoming the class clown or enticing others to join them in their off-task play. Still others may express their frustration through anger, striking out at those around them, because the real enemy—the disorder underlying their difficulties—cannot be hit or pushed or yelled at. When the need to strike out at something, anything, becomes overwhelming or frequent, these children may be labeled "behavior problems."

Some children do indeed exhibit true psychiatric disorders that result in destructive behaviors; nevertheless, it is important to recognize that we all need to release pressure by blowing our tops from time to time. Young children are no exception. But for the young child with a disorder such as APD, this frustration may become all-encompassing. Combine this with the exhaustion from having to try so hard to listen, to learn, to complete homework that should take no time at all, and it is not surprising that some children with APD are unable to cope and lash out violently with words or actions.

Expressing frustration with certain tasks, such as saying "I can't do this" or "I don't understand." Young children learn so many new skills so quickly that they often respond with frustration and the words "I can't . . ." However, when a child utters these words every time a particular type of task is required of her, we should begin to pay attention to the demands involved.

Most young children will approach new learning opportunities with an inner belief in their ability to succeed, if not a palpable excitement and eagerness. Sadly, if a child is confronted with repeated failure despite her best efforts, her excitement will dim and resistance will take its place. A child who automatically responds to every multistep direction with "I don't understand" even before the instructions are delivered or throws every book aside, saying "I can't do this" even before trying to read a single word, may be telling us precisely what kinds of difficulties she is having.

Demonstrating poor problem-solving skills. In the previous chapter, we discussed the relationship between auditory processing and many types of problem-solving. Children with APD may demonstrate difficulty with math word problems, devising communication repair strategies to overcome misunderstandings, predicting what comes next in a story, inferring outcomes based on causal factors, generalizing information learned to new problems and situations, and many other academic and social situations involving the ability to problem-solve. All of these activities require the child to comprehend all of the critical information, then apply it to the problem at hand. Anything that disrupts this complex flow, including any auditory disorder that impairs the acquisition of the information in the first place, will certainly have an effect on the child's ability to arrive at a solution.

Performing better when auditory information is augmented with visual or tactile cues. One of the most common, and frequently most effective, strategies to assist a child with an APD in learning new information is to present the information visually or to provide objects that can be manipulated to reinforce the concepts being taught. A child with an APD is often described as a "visual learner," one who learns best when material is presented through pictures and hands-on demonstrations. So, an important factor in determining whether a child may exhibit an APD is how well the child learns through other senses, such as vision. Logically, a child who has difficulties regardless of whether information is presented verbally, visually, or through hands-on demonstrations would not be considered to have a purely auditory disorder.

An important caveat must be issued here: For children with APD that involves inefficient interhemispheric integration, the addition of visual or hands-on cues may actually confuse rather than clarify the information presented, making their difficulties even more apparent. This is because interhemispheric disorders can lead to difficulty processing and integrating information from the different senses simultaneously. It should never be assumed that more is better. If multisensory cues seem to confuse the child, the possibility of an interhemispheric disorder should be considered.

The use of symptom checklists or key indicators may be helpful in determining whether a child has problems with auditory processing. Nevertheless, the heterogeneity of this disorder and the similarity of symptoms of APD to those of other disorders means that checklists such as these can neither be relied on exclusively nor used diagnostically.

I frequently receive communications from parents who have accessed similar checklists from Web sites or brochures on APD and who say, "I'm sure that my child has an APD because he fits *every one of these symptoms* exactly." I have also seen many children who were "diagnosed" with APD by a psychologist or physician or other professional on the basis of checklists such as the one presented in this section. Each of these symptoms manifests itself in complex ways, and each manifestation can represent different types of dysfunction in different parts of the brain. Many of these symptoms also "fit" other disorders, as well. For that reason, if a child appears to exhibit every one of these symptoms, I am far less likely to consider an APD as the key contributing factor to the child's difficulties than I would be if the symptoms fit some logical *pattern,* with some items being applicable and others not, that would be consistent with a particular type (or combination of types) of APD. For example, when a child exhibits behaviors consistent with left-hemisphere dysfunction, but does better in those areas associated with the right hemisphere, this makes far more sense from a neurophysiologic perspective than the child who exhibits a smattering of left-, right-, and interhemispheric symptoms. Furthermore, these logical patterns of behavioral symptoms will coincide with patterns in the results of diagnostic testing. Like pieces of a jigsaw puzzle, they allow us to arrive at an accurate diagnosis of the presence and nature of an APD and to develop treatment plans that will address the needs of the individual child. But, like a jigsaw puzzle, if some of the pieces are missing, it is impossible to construct a complete picture.

As we have seen, the presence of APD in elementary school can interfere with the child's ability to learn the basics upon which he will build in later grades, as well as with the ability to make friends and to be a kid. Often the first suspicion that an APD may be present arises in elementary school, because of the presence of key indicators of auditory processing difficulties. If diagnosed early, many of the learning and social deficits that accompany APD may be addressed and treated. That's why parents should bring up any concerns they may have about their child's learning or communication abilities to the teacher or appropriate other personnel at their school as soon as possible. The provisions of IDEA entitle every child to a "free and appropriate public education" (FAPE), including those children with disabilities. By law, if parents express in writing (or orally, in the case of parents who are unable to write) concern that their child may have a disability, the school system is required to look into the matter. The determination of the need for further evaluation, however, is a team decision. This team, comprising school- and special-education-related professionals and the parents, will collectively decide whether the child meets the requirements for a disability requiring special education services as defined by the particular state.

As the child moves from elementary school into middle and high school, the demands—both linguistically and socially—become ever more complex and difficult. Problems may emerge that were not seen in elementary school, as children who exhibited few (or even no) signs of a disorder in the earlier grades may suddenly begin to have difficulty.

PROM NIGHT: APD IN MIDDLE AND HIGH SCHOOL

Middle and high school can be a truly terrifying experience for the child with an APD. Gone is the comfort of having one teacher for every class. Children must now deal with changes not only in speakers, but also in listening environments, rendering classroom-based management of APD much more unwieldy. As upper grades are reached, more and more information is presented via lectures, posing new and ever more complex difficulties.

These factors, plus the unavoidable onset of puberty and the ever-increasing peer pressure, can result in an entirely new set of problems that require different solutions from those that were reasonable and effective during the elementary-school years. All of the key indicators presented in the previous section continue to apply to the adolescent or teenager with APD. They may be manifested, however, in different ways, due to changes in the environment, in the learning demands, and in the children themselves. Factors that were merely mild annoyances or perhaps even not apparent during the elementary-school years may become pivotal issues in upper grades.

One of the most apparent differences between elementary school and middle or high school is the learning environment itself. In elementary school, children usually spend the majority of the academic day in one classroom with one teacher, moving to other rooms and teachers only for such activities as computer lab, art, music, and gym. Some elementary-school children do go to other classrooms or teachers for certain subjects, such as math; however, these transitions are usually introduced gradually and orderly. Children may line up at the door and traipse en masse to another room for a specific subject, or to the cafeteria for lunch. When classroom modifications such as preferential seating or an assistive listening device are required because of a child's disability, these modifications can often be implemented rather easily, especially if there is minimal changing of rooms by the child. Routines are simpler in elementary school as each day is organized like all of the others.

All of this changes in middle school. Adolescents must change classrooms and teachers for each subject and do so independently, without the orderly line they may have become accustomed to in elementary school. Furthermore, in many schools, a student's schedule will change from day to day and week to week. Each classroom change means a change in seating arrangements, acoustic characteristics, classmates, and teacher styles. An elementary-school strategy adopted for a given classroom's characteristics or a given teacher's style may not be appropriate for the classes in middle or high school. Adolescents may have difficulties in academic subjects at which they previously excelled, simply due to changes in teachers or classrooms.

I once worked with a fourteen-year-old boy who exhibited a speech-sound-based APD first identified in elementary school. We had employed direct therapy techniques for Craig and had also implemented a variety of classroom management strategies. Some of these strategies included wearing an FM system (a listening device in which the microphone is worn by the teacher and the receiver is worn by the student to enhance the signal-to-noise ratio) and having Craig sit where he could see the teacher's face at all times. Like many children with this type of APD, Craig had the most difficulty with verbal-based subjects such as language arts, reading, and science. In contrast, he was a true whiz at math. Craig complained of great difficulty in hearing, especially in backgrounds of noise, and exhibited poor word-attack abilities in spelling and reading. Our intervention had consisted, in part, of specific therapy to help him learn to discriminate among speech sounds, to link the speech sounds with letters in reading and spelling, and to bolster related phonological awareness abilities. By the time Craig left elementary school for the local junior high school, he had improved remarkably in his ability to understand the material and instructions presented in class and in his reading and spelling skills, and his grades had skyrocketed because of it.

When Craig reached the seventh grade and entered junior high, he began to experience the same types of difficulties that he had shown in earlier grades. Reading and spelling became areas of concern, as did Craig's ability to understand what was being discussed or presented in lectures. Most surprising, however, was that he began to demonstrate difficulties in the one subject at which he had always excelled—math. And all of this despite his having an *individualized education plan (IEP)* in place. His IEP identified him as a student with a learning disability and set forth specific modifications and special education services, all of which were being followed to the letter at the new junior high school.

Craig and his parents returned to my clinic partway through the fall semester at his new school. They had vacillated between despair prior to his initial diagnosis, to hope following the diagnosis, to ecstasy when he had appeared to overcome his disorder. Now they were back to despair. It seemed as if all of the intervening years, all of Craig's hard work and the implementation of classroom modifications and strategies, had not even occurred. When I saw him this time, Craig was even more despondent than he had been at our first meeting.

Craig's auditory processing abilities had actually improved significantly over the years, as expected. Now, however, several factors were responsible for the resurgence of his difficulties. A multidisciplinary team approach was again required, and careful observation of the characteristics of every one of Craig's classes was also necessary. Some of Craig's apparent backslide could be attributed to class- or teacher-related issues, and some was a product of changes in Craig's behavior and priorities, in himself.

Craig had not been wearing his FM system in the classroom. He would forget to get the microphone from one teacher to the next. In addition, Craig's battery charger for his FM system was placed in the first room he attended in the morning. Because he was not required to return to that room anytime during the day, he would frequently forget to retrieve the microphone and charge it and his receiver overnight. So, his batteries were often dead, and most of the time the system didn't work.

Even when the FM system was working appropriately, Craig would feel self-conscious as he and his classmates watched their teacher hook the lapel mike to her collar and make any necessary adjustments. Something that had been done rather subtly by the elementary-school teacher had now become a ritual performed several times a day before an audience of Craig's classmates, which drew attention to his use of the device. Use of the FM system set Craig apart from the rest of the crowd, and for the first time in his life, he was embarrassed to be seen wearing it.

This reaction is not surprising considering the amount of peer pressure on adolescents. In fact, my experience has been that, even if a child willingly uses an assistive listening device during the elementary-school years, he may rebel against it once he reaches the age at which other kids' opinions become all-important. Preteens and young teenagers want to be like the rest of the kids—from the logo on their tennis shoes to the label on their jeans. And if they're not, they hear about it from the others. Something as small as not having the coveted item of the day could set a kid up for ridicule. The use of an FM device was a pretty obvious indicator that Craig was different. Through careful and gentle questioning, Craig revealed that some of the other kids had already begun to make fun of him because of it. In fact, he asserted in a rare moment of rebellion, he didn't want to use it anymore at all, even if it meant failing every subject.

Although his mother's initial inclination was to force Craig to continue to use the device for his own good, I actually agreed with Craig. Assistive listening technology can be helpful in providing clearer access to information that is presented in class, but for proper use it does require commitment on the part of the student and the teachers. Because the presence of an APD can interfere with socialization anyway, if the use of such a device results in social difficulties, insisting on its use may do more harm than good. Socialization and being accepted take precedence over academic achievement, at least to a preteen kid, so it is important to consider these changing priorities when recommending classroom interventions. For these reasons, we decided that Craig would no longer be required to use the FM device.

Not all of Craig's difficulties were due to his unwillingness to use his FM system. As expected, the linguistic level of the information presented in his classes was far higher than what he had been exposed to at his previous school. Also, the vast majority of the material was presented via lecture, with occasional visual aids or demonstrations in those classes—such as science—that lend themselves to these. Students were also expected to take notes. A system of "guided note-taking" had been implemented in the first few weeks, and by the middle of the semester students were expected to take good notes independently. To pass written exams on the material covered, students were expected to study these notes and the accompanying reading assignments and worksheets. Although Craig had continued to place himself in the most advantageous position in each of his classrooms—with easy visual access to the teacher and away from any sources of noise, such as radiators—he was having great difficulty in *listening* and *writing* simultaneously.

Note-taking requires a student to divide his attention, which can pose significant problems for a child with an APD. Even under ideal listening conditions and with full attention directed toward hearing and understanding lectures, students with APD often miss a great deal of information. When note-taking is required, the student is less able to devote attention to listening and will, therefore, miss even more of the information presented. Finally, note-taking requires the ability to extract the key points of a message and write them down.

Because many students with APD have difficulty extracting key points, writing, and spelling, note-taking may be much harder for a student with an APD than for a child without a disability. Note-taking may seem impossible for students with APD.

Essentially, for a child such as Craig, note-taking represents all of his most problematic areas tied up in one tidy bundle. Everything suffers. He hears less, understands less, writes less, and has fewer or poorer-quality notes to go on when studying for exams. The reading material is not much help as its linguistic level is quite high, and much of the material presented in the lecture is not included in the book. For Craig, walking into a written exam was much like the nightmare, which many of us have had at some point, of showing up at a test only to find that we have never learned the material in the first place. Only, for Craig, this was no nightmare. This was very real. The reason for the resurgence of Craig's difficulties in verbal-based subjects was quite clear, so one of the new classroom modifications implemented for him was to provide a note-taker so that he could focus his entire attention on hearing and understanding the lectures.

None of this, however, explained why Craig was having difficulty in math—a subject at which he had previously excelled. A visit to his classroom solved this mystery. Craig's math teacher was a wonderfully sweet woman, with a quiet, gentle voice and a true knack for explaining concepts clearly. Unfortunately, at times her voice was difficult to hear. Worse, however, was that Craig's math class was on the other side of the wall from the band room, and sure enough, eighth-grade band practice took place at the same time as Craig's math class.

Switching to a different math classroom or teacher was not an option for Craig. For a while, we were somewhat at a loss. But Craig came up with a solution himself. He suggested using the FM system again, but *only* during math class and *only* if the teacher promised to have the microphone on and ready to go before the students arrived. He himself would sit near the back of the room—where he could still see the teacher clearly but not feel as if he were on display. The battery charger would be kept in the math room as well, so that Craig could remember to recharge his unit every night. Finally, the math teacher would supplement her spoken lectures with written notes to be provided to Craig before class. In this way, Craig was able to take charge of his listening environment, independently arrive at a solution, and once again excel in his primary area of academic excellence.

I cannot overemphasize the importance of empowerment for any child with an APD. Children (and adults) with APD must be made to feel as if they have some power over their environment and their disorder. To this end, we will later discuss compensatory strategies that can be taught to children and adults to help them become active listeners and to take control of their own listening success. In Craig's case, that he was able to come up with a solution himself was so liberating that he didn't even pause to consider that he had done a 180-degree turn from his previous refusal to use assistive listening technology under any circumstances. This was *his* decision, and he was incredibly compliant and consistent in using the device. After all, it was his idea.

Craig's independent search for solutions to listening difficulties—what we call active listening behaviors—extended to other classes, as well. By the end of his first year in junior high school, he had become rather adept at what is referred to as scoping it out. He could evaluate a classroom setting in a snap, choose the place where he would have the most access to information and the least amount of distraction, and fill in gaps by consulting notes taken by others or clarifying with the teacher after class. Each new classroom or teacher required careful analysis and a plan of attack, a challenge that Craig came to view with relish, almost like solving a difficult puzzle or mystery. These independent skills and compensatory strategies served Craig well throughout his junior high years and well into high school.

We also continued with more advanced direct therapy techniques appropriate for adolescents, and Craig's auditory skills improved. Additional improvements in reading and written language abilities soon followed.

Craig's success was due in large part to his willingness, indeed his *eagerness,* to learn and succeed academically. But not all preteens and adolescents demonstrate such eagerness to learn. Where a small child might view learning as the unveiling of things heretofore mysterious and elusive, often much of the shine has rubbed off by the time he reaches middle school. It takes an unusual maturity for a teen to really see that learning is important for the future. Most teens are far more concerned with how well they are accepted by others. For an adolescent or teenager to actually *choose* to comply with suggestions for learning that may set him apart from the rest goes against the prime motivating factors at this age. What teen would choose to practice at-home therapy techniques over going to a school dance or participating in after-school sports? What teen would wear a funny-looking thing on her head or ears after she had taken so much care with her hair and earrings, not to mention her clothing? What teen would apply himself diligently to hours and hours of homework every night, knowing all the while that his friends have already finished and are watching championship wrestling on television? These are not trivial concerns. When working with middle and high school students with APD, we are dealing with very different motives and priorities from those that drive younger children. If we do not respect these priorities, we will be unlikely to effect changes that will ultimately help the child.

Children with learning difficulties or disorders such as APD may find themselves associating with, even embracing, activities and individuals that dismay their parents just for the right to say "I belong." In my practice, I have seen many high school students with APD who have engaged in delinquent behavior, including gang activity, truancy, drug use, and sexual promiscuity. Many of our juvenile correctional facilities are filled with teens who have learning disabilities or other disorders that affect their ability to communicate and learn.

While we might be able to understand why a child with a disability might, after years of struggle and failure, begin to rebel and act out, it is important not to attribute all of the behavioral difficulties the child exhibits to the disorder. For every child with an APD who engages in delinquent behavior, countless others continue to put forth good effort, actively participate in therapy and management activities, and meet expectations at home and at school. We must always be careful to distinguish between the disorder itself and the behaviors that overlie and sometimes sabotage the child's efforts to overcome the disorder.

Some psychiatric disorders affect a child's ability to distinguish between right and wrong (such as oppositional-defiant disorder and conduct disorder), but APD is not one of them. There is a vast difference between being *unable* and being *unwilling*. Some children with APD and related disorders may take control of their circumstances through denial, rebellion, and self-destructive behaviors; however, these are *choices* made by the child, not unavoidable outcomes imposed by the presence of the disorder.

High school students with APD face unique challenges in both learning and socially. How they choose to face these challenges will have a significant impact on how successful they are in overcoming their disorders. All of the key indicators of APD we have discussed continue to apply to adolescents and teens. In addition, middle and high school students with APD *may*

- Exhibit a reappearance of earlier complaints and symptoms or an entirely new set of difficulties because of the changing academic demands of higher grades

- Demonstrate difficulties in classes at which they had excelled previously due to classroom acoustics, differing teacher styles, or a host of other factors

- Have problems understanding concepts presented in lecture-based classes because of difficulty with note-taking and comprehending reading assignments

- Earn poor grades in foreign-language classes because of the new speech sounds and vocabulary that must be learned

- Exhibit difficulty with written tests, especially timed tests presented in multiple-choice or short-answer format, including college entrance exams

- Refuse to employ management strategies that will set the student apart from peers, such as the use of an assistive listening device, even if such strategies were complied with willingly in lower grades

- Withdraw from social communication or engage in self-destructive behavior; however, we must be careful not to attribute all undesirable behavior directly to the presence of an APD

The factors that affect adolescents and teens are far different from those in the elementary-school years, even if the disorder is the same. Therefore, strategies that were successful in addressing an elementary-school child's APD may no longer be effective in middle or high school. Entirely new intervention plans that take into account the child's new academic challenges and social-emotional priorities may need to be considered.

RUSH WEEK: APD AT COLLEGE

High school graduation may be the beginning of an exciting new life away from home for most young adults, but for those with APD the future contains an entirely new set of problems. Although they still have some legal rights that pertain to their disorder, college students with APD can no longer rely on the "free and appropriate public education" afforded them by federal law or many of the support services to which they have become accustomed. Nevertheless, they are still expected to demonstrate independence, academic achievement, and basic knowledge and skills beyond what was expected in high school. The most significant difficulty for a college student with an APD is the large classes conducted in lecture format. Depending on the size of the college, courses required in the freshman and sophomore years are typically taught in large lecture halls with often more than a hundred students in arena-style seating. To make matters worse, the acoustics in many older college classrooms are not always the best.

With the relatively recent surge in technology related to classroom acoustics and assistive listening devices, many of these lecture halls are now fitted with state-of-the-art microphone-and-speaker (sound-field) systems that really do provide for good clarity of the signal. But even in a classroom where such technology is in place, the student may feel that she is just an anonymous face in the crowd. Because much of the information will be presented via lectures, good note-taking skills are necessary, and the professor has little opportunity to ensure that each student understands the material presented. Imagine, if you can, the difficulty in standing for at least an hour every day in front of a room of a hundred or more students with a wide variety of skill levels and learning aptitudes, and teaching basic principles of psychology or earth science or English composition or any of a number of other courses. Even the best of professors cannot possibly monitor each student's face for signs of confusion. And even if that were possible, it would be difficult to attend to the needs of one student when ninety-nine or more other students in the same classroom may not share the same need for clarification.

A student with an APD will likely find this type of learning environment difficult, even if he has been doing well in smaller lecture-based classes in high school. Regardless of the type of APD, most students with APD will have difficulty because of the higher linguistic level of the material and the increased degree of independence expected of them. They will also have difficulty because of the increases in class size, workload, and reading assignments. Unfamiliar locations and teaching styles will also play a part in the problems students with

APD have with understanding the information, resulting in poor grades and frustration.

Even when students are able to learn the material presented, the way in which they are asked to demonstrate that knowledge may be far different in college. In high school, their grades may have been based in part on projects, take-home assignments, and written papers. In college, however, their grades will more likely be based on performance on two or three multiple-choice or short-answer written examinations. Students are expected to understand the material independently, integrate that material, understand the written questions on the exams, relate the questions to the learned material, and choose the correct answer(s). Students with difficulty in listening, note-taking, reading speed or reading comprehension, and so on will have difficulties with different parts of this overall process, but the results will be the same: poor grades on the exams and, therefore, poor course grades overall.

The teaching environment is not the only challenge facing a student with an APD. Once again, kids undergo a radical shift in priorities and behavior-related issues when the threshold to college is crossed. College-aged kids typically react in one of two ways when they experience their first sweet, exhilarating taste of independence. Some take it as an opportunity to buckle down and get on with learning. Others will take advantage of the fact that no one is present to tell them what they can or cannot do. Nevertheless, while the social dynamics of the college setting are far different from those of high school, socialization remains a priority for young college students.

It is not unusual for students with disabilities such as APD to find that their extracurricular activities have a more significant effect on their school performance than do those of other students. Most of us have schlepped into a classroom after pulling an all-nighter and tried to shake the fuzziness from our brains so that we can catch at least part of the lecture. But even on their best of days students with APD

must expend extra effort to obtain and understand verbally presented information. Anything that affects their ability to concentrate, especially the two most common factors that plague college
students—fatigue and poor nutrition—can leave them with few resources upon which to draw for learning in the classroom. Unfortunately, the normal activities associated with the college experience
may, themselves, lead to difficulties obtaining the most from that college experience.

I have worked with several college students—usually freshmen or
sophomores—who are having a great deal of difficulty in their college
classes. Many of these youths either did relatively well in high school
or had received special education services that assisted them daily in
learning. Although some had occasional or mild difficulties with paying attention or getting it in high school, these difficulties didn't really
interfere with their learning. In college, however, the unique characteristics of the setting, combined with the lack of someone to assist
them in the learning process, resulted in sudden, unexpected (and for
some students, disconcerting) academic difficulties, despite their putting forth effort equal to or greater than that expended by their peers.
Sometimes, the presence of a mild APD may not be identified until
problems surface in college. At other times, a known APD or a similar
learning disorder may need to be reconfronted and readdressed in
light of the new learning environment and the challenges unique to
the college setting.

Sometimes, the sudden appearance of academic difficulties in a
college-aged student may be attributed to "goofing off," partying too
much, or not having enough self-discipline to independently monitor
his own learning. This may be true in some cases. However, the presence of a possible disorder that was previously undiagnosed should be
considered in any student who appears to be putting forth good effort
with little success or who complains of difficulty hearing or understanding in the classroom. It's important to recognize what types of
learning difficulties a college student with an APD may experience.

But it's equally important to realize that students may have difficulties learning at college for many reasons that are not related to a disability or disorder. The language and concepts presented in college classes are far more advanced than those that were taught in high school, and some students arrive at college ill-prepared for these new academic demands. Others may find that they are unable to direct their own learning or that the amount of homework and reading is overwhelming. Many students fail to achieve high grades in college, even if they were A or B students in high school. Nevertheless, college students with APD *may*

- Complain of difficulty hearing or understanding lectures (particularly in very large classes, classes with poor acoustics, or with professors who speak rapidly), yet perform better in classes that are less lecture-oriented, such as science laboratories or mathematics

- Have significant difficulty taking notes during class and find it helpful to borrow notes from other students to guide them

- Demonstrate significant scatter in academic achievement, with poor grades in courses that rely on reading, listening, or understanding verbally presented concepts despite putting forth good effort

- Report that homework takes them far more time to complete than it does for peers in the same class

- Have a history of subtle difficulties in reading, spelling, comprehension, or related skills that become much more apparent after entering college

- Carry a previous diagnosis of APD or learning disability

- Exhibit extreme difficulty learning a foreign language or in other classes where most of the vocabulary is unfamiliar

- Have difficulty completing tests when a limited time is allowed, but do better when tests are untimed

- Obtain poor grades on certain types of tests (e.g., multiple-choice, short-answer), despite being able to demonstrate adequate understanding when allowed to respond orally

These are just some of the characteristics that a college student with an APD may exhibit. The presence of these behaviors and difficulties, however, does not mean that an APD is present. Only a careful, multidisciplinary assessment can determine whether a student's difficulties are due to an underlying disability.

The Americans with Disabilities Act (ADA) states that any individual with a physiologic disorder (which can include learning or communication disorders and APD) cannot be discriminated against in the educational arena, workplace, or other environments. For this reason, college students with disabilities are afforded certain rights that allow them the same access to education afforded to their nondisabled peers. Unlike IDEA, which provides every school-aged child with a free and appropriate public education and helps to ensure that each child *benefits* from such education, the provisions of ADA are concerned primarily with *access* and *discrimination* issues. If the individual has a disability that limits his access to the educational services, these access issues must be addressed by the educational institution. However, the responsibility for fulfilling job- or education-related expectations rests squarely on the individual.

Universities and colleges have disabilities services centers, offices designed to address education-related access concerns. The most obvious and familiar example of an accessibility issue is the wheelchair-bound student, who cannot be prevented from taking a course simply because the classroom is not accessible by wheelchair. However, the presence of an APD also may present accessibility concerns—specifically relating to access to verbally presented information in the classroom or even written information in exams and reading assignments. Even at the college level, support services such as the provision of a note-taker, more time to complete written exams, or tutoring services may be required for a student with an APD or related learning disabilities. Similar provisions may be required when taking standardized national examinations such as the Scholastic Achievement Tests (SATs) and Graduate Record Examinations (GREs).

Specific management suggestions for children and adults with APD will be discussed later; however, it is important to note here that the responsibility for compliance with many of these suggestions rests more heavily on the student when in college. During the school-aged years, children with disabilities requiring special education services have a specific plan of action developed, an individualized education plan (IEP). The IEP (or IFSP—individualized family services plan—for infants and children of preschool age), as required by IDEA, is essentially a contract drawn up by the teachers, administrators, special services providers, and parents that spells out precisely how a child's disability will be addressed in the educational setting. The IEP/IFSP includes specific goals, objectives, and activities, including classroom accommodations, that will allow the child to benefit from education. This is a team approach, and each team member has a responsibility to ensure that this contract is adhered to.

IEPs do not exist at the college level. In fact, even if a student is identified with a disability necessitating certain accommodations, there is no team meeting among all the professors and other individuals involved in the education of the student. Furthermore, the professors typically change from semester to semester, so it is entirely possible for a professor never to be aware that a student with a disability is in the class, especially when that disability is hidden, such as with APD or learning problems. It is the student's responsibility to inform every professor of his special needs, as well as to provide the appropriate supporting documentation to verify such needs.

Perhaps that, more than anything else, is the primary difference be-tween the high school and college settings, a difference that applies equally to personal and social pursuits and to learning. The college student is learning one of life's most important lessons: for the most part, he must look after himself rather than relying on others to act for him.

4

APD IN ADULTS

THE NOTION OF what constitutes a good listener changes as we become adults. The term takes on a more social connotation. Think, if you will, about the person whom you would consider a good listener. Is it the coworker who always has the right answer, carries out directions or instructions promptly, and always speaks when spoken to? Not likely. I would guess that it would be a friend who provides a shoulder to cry on, who nods at the appropriate moments, and who doesn't offer advice unless asked. As adults, sometimes the less we say or do, the better listeners we may seem to be. Children are expected to be active listeners who attend to, understand, and respond to the speaker appropriately. But good listening is often much more passive for adults. In many situations, just being there and nodding at the right moments is enough.

This shift in expected behavior means that listening disorders may become more difficult to detect in adults. Moreover, disorders such as APD may much more easily be hidden in adult life. We no longer have teachers or professors asking us point-blank questions or regularly requiring us to demonstrate our reading, writing, and comprehension skills. Depending on our work, we may even be able to nod and smile if we don't understand something that is said to us and still do the job—especially if that job involves repetitive, familiar tasks.

It's easy to see why APD in the adult population is so frequently overlooked. Unfortunately, even when APD is suspected or diagnosed, it is often dismissed as insignificant. This is hardly surprising. After all, which seems more important: APD in a young child who is learning how to talk, read, spell, and learn, or APD in an adult who has had those opportunities and is getting on with living?

Certainly, children with APD grow up to be adults with APD, and they must learn how to contend with aspects of the disorder in the workplace and at home. However, the most recent research into auditory processing and aging has shown that APD may accompany normal aging and it may occur at younger ages than we had ever imagined. APD can also result from brain injury in either children or adults. My own auditory processing problems, for example, were not caused by normal aging, but by an auto accident when I was in my midtwenties. Whatever the cause of APD in adults, its impact on an adult can be every bit as devastating as on a child. However, although the symptoms of APD remain much the same, it affects the daily life of an adult in different ways from that of a child.

We know that, as we age, many of us experience a decline in our vision and our hearing, as well as in other sensory and motor systems. We don't move as fast, hear or see as well. For some of us, our brains don't seem as sharp as they once did. In others, actual cognitive disorders such as Alzheimer's disease may occur. These changes happen earlier for some people than for others, but even those of us in our thirties or forties may be aware of subtle changes in the ways in which our bodies and minds function.

Searches for the causes of Alzheimer's, multiple sclerosis, Parkinson's disease, and other adult-onset disorders are ongoing. And while science has not yet been able to explain fully the cause of many of these, clearly their prevalence (including disorders that are considered part of normal aging) is on the rise. The reason for this is simple: the number of older adults is at an all-time high.

In response to the aging of the baby boomers, research on aging has dramatically increased. Some scientific findings have already helped to shed light on many of the difficulties aging adults experience in their everyday lives. Products designed specifically for aging adults are being marketed in magazines, newspapers, and on the television and radio.

Because so many older adults have hearing problems, hearing aid sales have never been so good and will only continue to increase in the upcoming decades. Furthermore, the technology used in those hearing aids has been improved in recent years to better address the types of listening problems that older people experience. Adults are becoming more educated and aware of the various problems facing them as they age. They are also becoming more knowledgeable about methods of prevention by keeping their bodies and minds in shape, and of technologies available to assist them in compensating for disorders they are experiencing.

Most exciting, perhaps, is the recent research into brain plasticity and aging. This research indicates that, through stimulation, we can actually improve the function—or slow the rate of degeneration—of the aging adult's brain. Although the brain is most plastic (or changeable) in young childhood, we now know that this neuroplasticity is not limited to the very young, as we once thought, but extends throughout the life span. Just as physical exercise can improve motor and range-of-motion function in the body (and defend against heart disease, high blood pressure, and osteoporosis), it also appears that exercising the mind can help to keep that critical organ in shape, too.

There has never been a more exciting time to be involved in aging research. It is important to recognize, however, that aging is not confined to the over-fifty crowd. Indeed, many disorders prevalent in the elderly are now thought to present themselves at much younger ages. Certainly, my own and others' research into auditory processing and aging has shown this to be true. In fact, for some people, auditory processing abilities begin to decline by age thirty-five or forty, a decline that may help to explain some of the communication difficulties we may have experienced in our spouses, friends, or even ourselves.

HE NEVER LISTENS ANYMORE: APD IN MIDDLE-AGED MEN

I can't count the number of times I have heard complaints like these from concerned, frustrated spouses: "He never listens to me anymore. I tell him to pick up milk at the grocery store, and when he comes home empty-handed, he swears I never mentioned it. I ask which dress he likes better—the red or the black—and he just smiles and nods. He turns the television up too loud, and when he's watching it, I could talk until I'm blue in the face and he acts like I haven't said a word."

Of course, the frustration becomes greater when hearing acuity is normal and no obvious reason for this relatively sudden listening difficulty can be found. Because we couldn't find an obvious hearing-related deficit to account for these behaviors, and because APD was a term typically applied to children, these listening problems in adults were once referred to collectively as *obscure auditory dysfunction*. More recently, however, we have begun to acknowledge that adults suffer from the same types of APD that occur in children. That is why we now use the term *auditory processing disorder* to refer to these deficits in everyone, regardless of age.

However, some in the field of aging and hearing argue that these age-related changes in listening abilities are not due to APD, but rather to changes in the inner ear that cannot yet be detected by our present diagnostic techniques. I, however, disagree, as do many other researchers in the field. We have uncovered evidence of auditory processing difficulties in aging adults that cannot reasonably be attributed to changes in the ear itself. These include shifts in right- versus left-hemisphere specialization for certain tasks, interhemispheric integration deficits, and deficits in processing fine time-related (or temporal) aspects of the speech signal. For example, we have shown that older listeners with normal hearing don't show the expected left-hemisphere specialization for certain speech sounds, which may account for their difficulty in being able to hear these speech sounds clearly. To make matters worse, the two hemispheres of the brain don't seem to work together as well as we get older. This can lead to problems with hearing speech in noisy backgrounds, linking the language of a message with tone-of-voice cues, and a host of other listening difficulties. And because the sounds of speech occur very rapidly, the temporal processing deficits seen in older adults can interfere with their ability to hear and understand. When we combine these factors with the hearing loss that often accompanies aging, it is no wonder that so many elderly adults have listening difficulties.

Changes occur in the entire auditory system, from the ear to the brain, as a result of the aging process. Like the chicken and the egg, it may be impossible to separate all brain-related changes from ear-related changes; however, it appears that some of the age-related degeneration that occurs in the central auditory system cannot be attributed to hearing loss or other ear-based pathology or dysfunction.

There are also gender differences in listening. Recent research into language processing in the brain, conducted by Drs. Joseph Lurito and Michael Phillips of the Indiana School of Medicine, has unveiled some amazing findings regarding brain function in men versus women. The researchers used magnetic resonance imaging (MRI) to study the brain activity of men and women listening to passages from a popular book. They found that, for men, listening-related brain activity was focused exclusively in the left (or dominant) hemisphere. Women, on the other hand, also demonstrated activity in the right hemisphere of the brain while listening. Thus, men appear to listen with only one side of their brain and women appear to use both.

Although this research is still preliminary, these findings may help to explain why left-hemisphere injury or stroke is typically much more destructive to language function in men than in women. They may also help to explain some of the differences between the genders in many communication-related areas, as well as providing insight into well-publicized observations that women typically are better than men at multitasking and performing other activities that require both sides of the brain to work together.

Research into differences in brain structure between men and women also suggests that some regions of the corpus callosum—the fiber tract connecting the two halves of the brain—are larger in women than in men. Moreover, some evidence indicates that age-related atrophy of this structure occurs earlier in men than in women. Changes in this region may occur in men by their late twenties, but not until the postmenopausal years in women.

Given this evidence, it seems logical that problems with listening activities that rely on these brain structures might occur at different ages for men than for women. Furthermore, these deficits might lead to different types of communicative difficulties for men than for women. Indeed, that is precisely what my own research has shown.

A large proportion of the adults who have come to me for assessment because of difficulties hearing, especially in noisy environments, are men in their late thirties or early forties. Almost without exception, they complain of having a hard time catching what is being said either in the workplace or at home. Sometimes, they deny the existence of a hearing problem, saying instead that the problem is that their wives insist on talking to them when they are washing dishes, running water, watching television, or at some other time when their attention is focused elsewhere. When questioned, most of these men concede that they do, indeed, feel as if they have a hearing loss, but that it is most noticeable when there is background noise. I refer to this phenomenon as "I can't hear you when the water's running."

Although this is a common complaint (especially for people with hearing losses that affect the higher pitches where many of the consonant sounds of speech occur), most of the men I see with this complaint do not exhibit any evidence of hearing loss whatsoever. Instead, my testing often indicates decreased interhemispheric integration, especially the inability to listen to two different signals at the same time.

In a comprehensive study of auditory processing abilities in normal men and women aged twenty to seventy-five, I found that men from thirty-five to forty exhibited significantly poorer auditory processing abilities than women of the same age. These men's difficulties related directly to how the two hemispheres of the brain interacted. Men from age twenty to twenty-five performed the same as women of those ages. Therefore, it appears that men begin to demonstrate difficulties in auditory processing earlier than do women. Not surprisingly, my study showed that men begin to demonstrate these difficulties at precisely the ages men begin complaining of difficulties hearing in noise.

Bryce was forty-two years old when I first met him. Although he described himself as a fun-loving guy with a large circle of friends, he was anything but gregarious when he arrived. Clearly, Bryce did not want to be at the clinic, having his hearing tested on a sunny spring afternoon. He carried a light windbreaker, which he twisted repeatedly in his fists as we were talking. Most of my questions were answered with monosyllabic answers. Bryce seemed embarrassed, almost apologetic, at having his communication difficulties exposed.

Bryce's wife, Cheryl, on the other hand, was as talkative as they come. I suspected that she was the primary force behind Bryce's visit, a suspicion that was confirmed when I asked Bryce, "So, what brings you here today?"

Bryce replied, somewhat dryly, "My wife."

"Actually, that's true," Cheryl said. "We came in my van, and no one drives the van but me."

"Are you having difficulty hearing?" I asked, knowing that he must be, else why would he be here?

"Nope. Well, *she* thinks I am," he amended grudgingly.

"Well, what types of hearing problems does *your wife* say you have?"

"I don't know. She says she tells me stuff that she never said and then gets mad when I don't remember."

"That's not it," Cheryl said earnestly. "I *do* tell him stuff, but he never listens anymore. Last week, I told him that Charles—that's our youngest son—that Charles had a parent-teacher conference at three in the afternoon and we were both supposed to go. He agreed he'd be there."

"I never agreed. How could I agree when you never told me?" Bryce protested.

"Well, you nodded," Cheryl pointed out shortly. "Same thing." She turned her attention back to me. "Anyway, there I am at the school with the teacher. Three o'clock comes and goes. No Bryce. It was really embarrassing. We went on without him because there were other parents waiting, but still . . ."

"You never told me about the meeting. I would have been there if you had," Bryce insisted once again.

"I did tell you and you nodded."

"Then I forgot," Bryce said, a slight edge surfacing in his voice. "Besides it was just that one time . . ."

"You always forget. And it happens all the time lately. It doesn't matter what I say, you never hear me, you don't listen. I could tell you the house is burning down and you'd probably just nod and go on with whatever it is you're doing."

Although Bryce and Cheryl had managed to keep their respective tones more or less on the light side during this rather entertaining exchange, I could sense a palpable undercurrent of frustration on both sides that suggested this wasn't the first time they had had this argument.

Bryce continued to defend himself: "Well, if you wouldn't always tell me stuff when I'm in the middle of doing something, I might be able to hear you better. You always decide to talk to me just when I get started with something."

Aha! I thought. "Bryce, what were you doing when Cheryl told you about the conference?" I asked.

"I don't know, I don't remember her telling me about it," Bryce replied, exasperated now.

"He was washing dishes," Cheryl said with certainty. "It was right after breakfast. He was washing, I was drying, and I told him like five times that the conference was that afternoon at three. And he *nodded*," she finished, fixing Bryce with a glare as she did so.

Over the next few minutes, we identified several situations in which Bryce had noticed difficulty hearing. In all of them there was background noise—from washing dishes to cocktail parties to shopping at the mall on a weekend afternoon. Bryce seemed best able to hear and understand what was being said when a room was quiet. But Bryce felt that he sometimes missed what was said when he didn't devote his full attention to listening, such as when he was concentrating on work-related papers. He worked in a sales office for a large computer manufacturer and hadn't really noticed much difficulty hearing at work. However, he did report that he sometimes had to ask clients to repeat themselves when he was conferencing with them on the phone and others in the office were talking at the same time. Even listening to a favorite television program while the kids were playing in a nearby room was frustrating for him, he revealed. Bryce seemed relieved to finally get all of this out in the open now that he had admitted a possible hearing problem.

Still, it remained to be determined why he was having these difficulties.

Standard hearing testing revealed Bryce exhibited completely normal hearing acuity in both ears. However, consistent with many men I have seen of Bryce's age with similar complaints, central auditory assessment indicated that he had difficulty attending to one ear and ignoring competing messages delivered to the other ear. He also found it hard attending to and repeating disparate information given to both ears at the same time. In addition, Bryce had difficulty verbally labeling patterns of tones that differed in pitch or duration (such as high-high-low or long-short-long)—which requires both halves of the brain to work together. He was, however, easily able to hum or mimic the tonal patterns presented because humming doesn't require the same type of interhemispheric cooperation that labeling does.

All of this suggested Bryce had a deficit in the interhemispheric integration of auditory information. That is, his hearing acuity was fine, but he had an APD, which I suspect was brought on by normal aging. At the ripe old age of forty-two, Bryce appeared to be a classic example of age-related APD.

I got to know Bryce and Cheryl quite well during the next several weeks. Because Bryce had little difficulty at work, most of our attention was focused on determining ways to manage Bryce's APD at home. Cheryl had to get Bryce's attention before giving him critical information. Bryce had to learn not to nod if he didn't hear something because, as Cheryl pointed out, nodding implied that he had both heard and agreed with what was said. To compensate for his disorder, Bryce learned to repeat or paraphrase what was said to him so that any misunderstandings could be corrected as soon as they occurred. He also kept a notepad with him to write down key information that needed to be remembered, such as appointments or grocery lists. The entire family made sure that the television was turned down or the water was shut off during important conversations. Family members and significant others should always be involved in counseling and management so that everyone understands and helps with overcoming the disorder.

Not all men of Bryce's age will exhibit APD. Nor is APD confined to men; women may have adult-onset APD for a variety of reasons, as well. Hearing loss may also be a contributing factor to listening difficulties even in young adults. In my practice, I see many adults with early-onset hearing loss, usually due to noise exposure. I live in an area with many farmers and industrial factory workers—noisy occupations. In addition, one of the most popular leisure activities in this area is hunting, a key cause of noise-induced hearing loss. When proper ear protection is not used, significant hearing loss can result from these occupational and leisure activities, resulting in listening difficulties similar to those seen in APD. Although there is no evidence to suggest that the noise exposure from such activities as listening to loud music, farming, or hunting causes APD, it can and does cause hearing impairment. And if a hearing loss exists, it will certainly combine with any APD that is present, leading to greater difficulty than with either disorder alone.

Bryce's listening problems were confined, for the most part, to home life and social situations. But APD can also cause difficulties in the workplace. For some, these difficulties may be no more than a mild annoyance—missing a word here or there, minor misunderstandings that inconvenience or harm no one. But for others, the problems that APD can cause at work are quite serious, indeed.

I once worked with an emergency dispatcher for an inner-city police station who had adult-onset APD. In an area where gang-related shootings, stabbings, and other crimes were rampant, his job was to get the details quickly from callers and to relay them to mobile units so that they could respond. He was one of several dispatchers working in a noisy radio-communications room. To make matters worse, most of the callers were in panic, talking rapidly and often in noisy environments themselves. As my patient's APD worsened, he found himself having to ask for repetitions more frequently, and he lived in fear that he would get the details wrong and cost someone his life. Thankfully, this never happened, but his fears were justified. Lives did indeed depend on his ability to hear the facts clearly and accurately. We tried several types of technology to make the incoming signal clearer, and we plugged his free ear so that the noise from the communications room would be less of an interference. Despite all of our efforts, however, he continued to feel that his APD was a significant liability. He prudently removed himself from that job and requested reassignment to another, less auditorily challenging, position in the department.

In countless other cases, however, we have successfully treated or compensated for APD in the work setting. I have helped lawyers and judges with APD to be successful listeners in the courtroom with a little assistance from hearing technology and training in methods of compensation. Dentists, firefighters, teachers, and salespeople have overcome their auditory disorders and continued on in their chosen careers. For every person who must face the need to change job settings because of an APD, many others learn to overcome the disorder and succeed at work. We will talk about specific methods of coping with APD in the workplace later. But it is important to understand that, with cooperation from family, friends, coworkers, and supervisors, most adults with APD can lead successful, productive, and satisfying personal and professional lives.

I JUST CAN'T SAY ANYTHING RIGHT: APD IN POSTMENOPAUSAL WOMEN

Rose was a fifty-nine-year-old woman who looked half that age. She was well educated, with a master's degree in library science and a doctorate in English literature. She worked from home as an editor and researcher for authors, particularly those specializing in historical fiction.

Rose was not referred to me because of any listening difficulties. Her hearing seemed to be just fine and she had no auditory complaints whatsoever. What brought Rose to my office was a conversation I had had with a good friend of mine, an obstetrician/gynecologist. We had been discussing my recent findings regarding auditory processing and postmenopausal women, and he had said, "Wow, I have a lady I'd really like you to meet. It would be interesting to see what her testing showed."

Rose had recently gone through menopause, a change that she had been well prepared for, having independently researched the condition at the first signs of menstrual irregularity and hot flashes in her late forties. She had anticipated virtually all of the physical and emotional changes that would occur. However, nothing had prepared Rose or her husband for the difficulties they began to experience in their relationship. Rose had always prided herself on her internal control, her calm in the face of any crisis. Now, however, she found herself overreacting to the smallest of things—an inappropriate or insensitive tone of voice, a perceived slight from a family member or friend. She had expected some degree of increased emotional lability with menopause, but this was far beyond the realm of what she considered normal.

By the time I saw Rose, she and her husband, Richard, were in marital therapy with a psychologist specializing in couples and relationships. Rose and Richard had had a stable relationship for more than twenty-five years, and they had seen each other through the rearing of three children, Rose's education, Richard's change of occupation from corporate manager to independent consultant, and his bout with testicular cancer ten years previously. Their marriage had weathered many storms, but now it seemed as if it might, inconceivably, be winding to an end.

Rose felt that their ability to talk openly with one another had undergone a change that had coincided with her own change of life. For example, she stated that, whereas Richard always had treated her with the utmost respect and had patiently and respectfully listened to her views throughout their marriage, he had recently begun to patronize her and cut her off abruptly. In fact, Rose asserted, he seemed to be laughing or sneering at her every time she set forth any opinion, from the color of the kitchen wallpaper to current political affairs. Alternatively, he responded so abruptly he clearly didn't want to hear what she had to say at all. This man with whom she had shared so much seemed suddenly to disdain her very presence. Even worse, something was often in his tone that suggested he was hiding something. She couldn't quite put her finger on it, but a tiny suspicion had begun to form in Rose's mind that Richard might be having an affair. Rose suspected that menopause, for which she had been so prepared, had somehow robbed her of her femininity in Richard's eyes, had made her less attractive to him.

For his part, Richard seemed confused and bewildered. He vehemently denied having an affair or even considering one. He stressed again and again that Rose was just as attractive, as beautiful inside and out, as she had been the very first time he had set eyes on her. Richard still desired her and considered her his best friend. She was and always had been the only woman for him. He felt Rose was reacting strangely, that everything he said was misconstrued. He had always had a rather sardonic wit, he said, and Rose had always appreciated his sense of humor. Now, however, she took everything literally and reacted emotionally to even the most innocuous of comments. Richard was emotionally exhausted. "I just can't say anything right," he said.

Rose's physician and the psychologist working with the couple both felt that Rose's emotionality was far beyond what would be expected from hormonal issues alone. Searches for alternative explanations— long-standing repressed marital problems that were just now coming to the forefront; changes in Rose's perception of herself as a desirable woman being projected onto Richard—had failed to reveal any hidden cause for their sudden difficulty. Both standard psychotherapy and marital counseling were ineffective. Rose and Richard defended their separate positions and views with conviction, and each seemed sincere in his or her perception of the other's behavior. After several months of counseling, they were at an impasse.

At this point, Rose's physician suggested that I see her. Rose arrived at my office somewhat skeptical. She held little hope that an audiologist such as myself could provide any illumination of her marital difficulties when those professionals who specialized in marital discord had failed. Nevertheless, she was willing to undergo my tests and answer my questions on the off chance that some tiny nugget of evidence might emerge to help explain her difficulties.

For my part, I was skeptical, too. I am an audiologist, not a marriage counselor. The difficulties that Rose and Richard were having were far outside my scope of practice, and I did not feel qualified to address them in any way. Despite my research into auditory processing in postmenopausal women, I thought we were grasping at straws here. But I, like Rose, was interested in what we might find. And I trusted my friend, Rose's physician, when he asserted confidently that the types of auditory difficulties my research had found in some post-menopausal women just might provide an explanation for Rose's complaints. The similarities between Rose's complaints and my personal experiences with right-hemisphere-based auditory processing difficulties (especially the effects my own disorder had had on communication with my husband) provided further justification for Rose's tests.

Rose's test results suggested that she did, indeed, exhibit an auditory processing deficit, one that I had come to associate with some postmenopausal women and with APD involving the right hemisphere of the brain. In fact, Rose's pattern of findings on these tests precisely mirrored my own: She couldn't repeat information presented to her left ear when different information was simultaneously being given to her right ear. She couldn't hear subtle differences in pitch and duration of tonal patterns. But Rose's deficits in these areas were far more significant than what I had seen in my research study of normal adults. Auditory electrophysiologic testing also showed decreased activity on the right side of Rose's brain—further evidence that she exhibited a right-hemisphere-based APD, and a severe one, at that.

Although Rose may have had these difficulties long before she came to see me, that her communicative complaints were relatively new suggested that this was not the case. I cannot say for certain that menopause brought on these changes in auditory function, but nothing else in Rose's history coincided with her communicative difficulties—no illness, head trauma, hearing loss, or any other event or change in her life. Further neurologic and magnetic resonance imaging (MRI) evaluations of Rose subsequent to my findings also failed to uncover any other physiologic cause for her difficulties.

Following my testing, I became a team player in the counseling effort with Rose and her husband, which proved to be another example of multidisciplinary collaboration at its best. A good deal of the inter-

vention now consisted of increasing both Rose's and Richard's understanding of Rose's auditory perceptual difficulties, as well as methods
of compensating for such difficulties. I was able to share some of my
own personal insights and strategies that had worked for me under
similar circumstances—such as asking questions to clarify the intent
of others' communications, taking a breath before reacting negatively
to a perceived slight, and considering other possible meanings in addition to the ones that seemed obvious. We also undertook some direct therapy techniques focusing on melodic (pitch and duration)
discrimination, acoustic contour recognition, and interpretation of
verbal and nonverbal prosody cues. Because Rose and Richard now
had something to focus on—the auditory processing deficit rather
than some invisible and malevolent force intent upon disrupting their
marriage—they found that they were once again able to communicate
openly with each another. In fact, at one point, they stated that their
communication was perhaps even more open than it had been before,
because they had now become much more aware of not just *what* they
said to each other, but *how* they said it. Both of them felt as if they had
become more considerate and empathetic communicators, both in
their relationship with each other and with friends and acquaintances.

Since my experience with Rose and Richard, I have seen a number
of other women with virtually identical complaints. Some were seen
for routine hearing assessment and their communication difficulties
were revealed during the normal history-taking process. Others were
additional referrals from my friend, the OB-GYN, because of similarities in presentation to Rose. I suspect, however, that many women are
left untreated because they are not seen to have "auditory" difficulties
and, therefore, a referral to an audiologist such as myself would not
seem logical.

My research into auditory processing and aging has provided some
possible answers for why Rose, and women like her, may have these
types of auditory difficulties. I found that women, like men, tend to

exhibit decreased interhemispheric processing skills with aging. However, unlike men, the decrease in these processing skills occurs later in life—around the time of menopause. My research indicates that women in the immediate postmenopausal years (i.e., ages fifty-five to sixty) demonstrate the poorest auditory processing abilities of any age group, male or female, perhaps due to the wildly fluctuating hormonal changes in play at that time in a woman's life. These women were also the only ones to exhibit deficits in the perception of tonal patterns— or acoustic contours—which we associate more with right-hemisphere dysfunction than with interhemispheric dysfunction. It appears that women in the immediate postmenopausal years may have a harder time reading tone-of-voice cues that convey the underlying, sometimes hidden, meaning of speech. Because of this, these women may be unable to judge what a person really *means* in relation to what he or she *says*.

Other research I have completed suggests that the brain representation of speech sounds, as measured by auditory electrophysiology, is less active over the left hemisphere (and more active over the right hemisphere) in women older than fifty-five. When taken together, these findings led me to hypothesize that women in the postmenopausal years may exhibit different types of communication difficulties than those exhibited by men. Men tend to complain more of hearing-in-noise difficulties and problems hearing precisely what was said. Postmenopausal women may have more difficulty determining the hidden meaning of conversations, appreciating subtle aspects of humor and sarcasm, and exhibit other misperceptions related to what is *meant*. Some of the "emotional lability" of peri- and postmenopausal women might, indeed, be due to auditory perceptual difficulties.

From an evolutionary and biological perspective, these changes make sense. Females in the human and animal kingdom need to maintain sharp auditory perceptual skills throughout the childbearing years. They need to, for example, respond to their offsprings' needs while, at the same time, listening for predators. Subtle changes in pitch or rhythm of their offsprings' vocalizations might signal entirely different needs. Therefore, females may retain this ability until menopause, when the childbearing and child-rearing years typically come to an end. Males, on the other hand, do not have such dual responsibilities, at least from the perspective of survival of the species.

Once again, a caveat is in order here. My research results provide merely the first inkling of the possibility that, for some women, APD may be a contributing factor to communication difficulties in the postmenopausal years. This area needs much more study and systematic research before any firm conclusions can be drawn. In addition, auditory processing and communication abilities are merely one small part of the intricate web of interpersonal relationships during the menopausal years or at any point in life. Just as we cannot attribute all language and learning problems in children to APD, we cannot and should not think that all relationship difficulties, even those that appear to be communicative in nature, are due to APD. Finally, we must realize that menopause is a dramatic life event that, combined with hormonal changes, can and does lead to increased emotionality in many women. To even attempt to suggest that all of the difficulties in the emotional and communication domains that women of this age experience might be due to APD would be indefensible.

However, it appears that some women do exhibit changes in auditory processing during menopause, and these changes may affect their ability to understand the intent of others' communications. Further, preliminary data suggest that this difficulty may be more pronounced in women who are not undergoing estrogen supplementation. This is consistent with other findings indicating that hormonal replacement therapy may have an effect on other aspects of cognition, as well. Further research is needed to explore this phenomenon more fully, as well as to determine effective and appropriate means of treating and managing these types of disorders from a multidisciplinary perspective. We also need to focus on ways of helping men and women understand the communication difficulties of the opposite gender. Everyone needs to be better informed of the unique communication difficulties that may arise from adult-onset APD.

EVERYBODY'S MUMBLING AT ME: APD IN THE ELDERLY

A decrease in hearing acuity is one of the most common effects of aging. A lifetime of noise exposure, genetic predisposition, and a variety of physical changes cause most elderly people to experience some degree of hearing loss. Age-related hearing loss, termed *presbycusis,* is usually characterized by poorer hearing for higher frequencies or pitches. This type of hearing loss can make some speech sounds harder to hear than others. Many of the consonant sounds of speech, *t* and *s* for example, are quiet and higher in frequency and, thus, more difficult to discern. In contrast, the lower-pitched vowel sounds, which carry much of the "loudness" or energy of speech, are often heard just fine. One of the most common complaints of elderly listeners is that although speech may sound loud enough (or even, in some cases, too loud), they still have a difficult time actually understanding what is said. Furthermore, when the speaker shouts (a natural but rarely productive tendency), the only result is annoyance on the part of the elderly listener, as speech just becomes louder, not clearer.

Presbycusic hearing loss often leads the elderly to state, "Everyone seems to be mumbling." This makes sense when you consider that clear diction relies on precise production of the consonants—the very sounds that elderly listeners may have a difficult time hearing. This difficulty is more pronounced in backgrounds of noise, where the noise masks those frequency regions in which the elderly listener has better hearing, leaving him or her with little to go on. This happens even if the speech seems loud enough to hear quite well.

We have known about these changes for many decades now. We have also known that they can be attributed to damage in the hair cells of the inner ear. In other words, what the ear gives the brain to process is distorted or incomplete in elderly listeners with hearing loss. That's why ear-based changes in hearing acuity can lead to changes in the way the brain pathways process auditory information.

What is just becoming apparent, however, is that the listening problems of some elderly people cannot be accounted for by ear-related changes in hearing acuity alone. Ample evidence suggests that the brain pathways themselves change as a result of aging, and that some of these changes cannot be attributed to hearing loss. We have come to refer to the reduction in central auditory processing abilities with aging as *central presbycusis*—or aging-related APD.

Recent research has shown that one key difference between elderly and young listeners is the way in which the two hemispheres of the brain communicate with one another. Men may begin to show these interhemispheric processing difficulties in relatively early adulthood. These difficulties continue to decline progressively up to about age fifty-five or so. In contrast, the interhemispheric processing abilities of women seem to be relatively well-preserved until the post-menopausal years. Then, women show both interhemispheric and right-hemisphere-based processing problems. Right-hemisphere auditory skills, such as interpreting tone-of-voice cues, appear to recover in these women as they age further. Their interhemispheric skills, however, do not. Therefore, by approximately age seventy, men and women demonstrate similar auditory processing deficits in how the two hemispheres of the brain interact.

The ability of the two hemispheres to communicate with one another is important for a variety of two-eared (*binaural*) listening abilities, not the least of which is understanding speech in noisy backgrounds. The decrease that elderly men and women show in inter-hemispheric functioning contributes to their difficulties hearing in noise and to other binaural listening deficits. For those elderly people who do not have significant hearing losses, this may be the primary factor causing their listening difficulties.

This type of APD also appears to relate directly to how successful and satisfied an elderly person will be with hearing aids. When an elderly person shows signs of hearing difficulties, it is usually assumed that he or she needs a hearing aid—which, it should be pointed out, is often entirely true. And for most people, two hearing aids are better than one, because two can simulate the natural state of two-eared hearing that we are born with.

Recent advances in hearing aid technology have rendered these tiny devices truly remarkable in their clarity and quality. Nevertheless, hearing aids are not like glasses. With glasses, what you see is clear and natural as soon as you put them on—it is as if your normal vision were restored. Hearing aids, however, do not make sound completely clear and natural. Hearing aids rely on electronic circuitry, so there will always be some distortion. And although advances have been made in noise-reduction circuitry, hearing aids do tend to amplify unwanted sounds as well as desired speech. Speech-in-noise problems may persist even with the use of aids. This is why audiologists counsel listeners carefully about what they should realistically expect from hearing aid use. Two hearing aids are recommended more often because these will most closely mimic the normal state of two-eared hearing. Because listening with two ears is far better than having both the noise and the speech going into only one ear at the same time, binaural hearing aids will help listeners hear speech in noisy backgrounds better. But binaural hearing aids will not restore normal hearing in the same way that glasses seem to restore normal vision.

An elderly listener (or any hearing-impaired listener, for that matter) may reject hearing aids for many reasons. They might not like the constant visible reminder of their hearing loss or aging. They may be unwilling to admit that they have a hearing problem, preferring to believe that their difficulties arise from the "mumbling" of others. The hearing aid might be uncomfortable in the ear, or despite counseling about realistic expectations, it doesn't sound natural enough to them. The hearing aid may not be programmed correctly for their hearing loss. Unfortunately, rather than going through the sometimes tedious process of making minor adjustments to find the best settings for their particular listening characteristics, many people would rather just throw the darned thing in the trash and forget about it.

Sometimes, however, an elderly person may have an APD that is adding to the listening difficulties caused by hearing loss. When this happens, any auditory problems will be more pronounced than if either the APD or the hearing loss had occurred alone. And binaural hearing aids may just make matters worse. This was certainly the case with Ralph.

Ralph was seventy-two years old when he was first fit with hearing aids. Although his family had told him for years that he needed to have his hearing tested, he pooh-poohed their suggestions, insisting that he was just fine. Only after "constant badgering" (his words) by his daughter did Ralph agree to be seen by an audiologist. Hearing tests showed that Ralph had a rather typical hearing loss for a man his age and that his hearing was virtually identical in both ears. Ralph's hearing was worse in the higher frequencies, and he had some difficulty understanding speech, even in quiet situations. Ralph's ability to understand and repeat words improved significantly when the words were made louder so that he could hear more of the consonant sounds. But because he had relatively good hearing in the lower frequencies, he felt as though sounds were loud enough and had a difficult time understanding and accepting his need for amplification. Ralph didn't realize that hearing aids were not just designed to make sounds louder but could be programmed to enhance those frequencies where his hearing loss was greatest while minimizing amplification for those sounds he heard better. After quite a bit of discussion, including the assurance that the Consumer Protection Act allowed him to try hearing aids for thirty days before he had to pay for them, Ralph agreed— grudgingly—to give them a whirl.

Like most people with inner-ear hearing loss, Ralph exhibited a condition known as *recruitment* (abnormal loudness growth) that made him more sensitive to loud sounds. People with recruitment have a smaller-than-normal range between the point at which sounds can just barely be heard and the point at which they become uncomfortably loud. This limited dynamic range meant that Ralph's hearing aids needed to be programmed with circuitry that made sure that incoming sounds were not amplified beyond his uncomfortable-loudness level.

Ralph had hearing loss in both ears, so he would probably benefit most from two hearing aids. This was difficult for Ralph to accept. Hearing aids, which are usually not covered by insurance, can be quite costly. Two hearing aids means double the cost. Because Ralph was not at all enthused about wearing even one hearing aid, the thought of wearing two was even more onerous. The benefits of binaural hearing were explained to him. An analogy between glasses and hearing aids was made: You wouldn't wear a monocle rather than spectacles, would you? Reassurances were given that he could return one or both hearing aids if he wasn't satisfied. Finally, after a good deal of grumbling, Ralph agreed to try binaural amplification.

A week after Ralph was fitted for his hearing aids, he returned for some adjustments—with the aids in his pockets. "I don't like them," he said.

Ralph was not just being cantankerous. He had some very specific complaints. In particular, the hearing aids seemed to exacerbate Ralph's hearing-in-noise difficulties. Although he admitted that one-on-one conversation in quiet was a little easier, he reported that even the slightest presence of background noise made listening with the hearing aids unbearable. His daughter—hearing aid supporter that she was—admitted that Ralph did seem to communicate better in many situations without the aids than with them.

Adjustments were made to the programming circuits and Ralph was sent off once again to try the aids for another week. Once again, he was reminded of the need for consistent use of both aids.

A week later, Ralph returned with his daughter. Once again, his hearing aids rested in their cases in the pockets of his trousers. His daughter confirmed that he had tried, really tried, to comply with the recommendations and had worn the aids religiously for a couple of days or so. But to no avail. "They're driving me crazy," Ralph said with a good deal of frustration.

Again, more adjustments. Discussion about extending the trial period. Suggestions for trying different types or styles of hearing aids. Repeated counseling about realistic expectations. Another appointment for one week hence. This time, however, even Ralph's daughter seemed to view everything with skepticism.

The following week brought a surprise. Ralph arrived at the clinic with one hearing aid in place—the right one—and the other in his pocket. But the biggest surprise was the smile on his face. Triumphantly, he reached into his pocket, pulled out the leather case holding his left hearing aid, and handed it to the audiologist. "I'll take this one," he said, pointing to the aid in his right ear.

Ralph told how he had begun experimenting with the hearing aids over the past week. Initially reluctant, he had begun to view the aids as a puzzle to be solved or an adversary to be bested. Thus, he had worn both aids for two days, exposing himself to every situation under the sun—from the shopping mall to the local pub to the bingo hall, returning home only when he felt ready to scream with frustration. Then, he had worn just the left hearing aid for two days, repeating his previous actions with similar results. Finally, as a last resort, he had worn just the right aid, believing without a doubt that he would end up returning both of them and demanding a full refund at the end of the week. To his extreme surprise, not only was wearing the right aid tolerable, he actually liked it. With a proud grin, he reported how he experienced a significant improvement in his listening and understanding abilities when using the hearing aid in just his right ear. Of course, he said, it wasn't perfect—it still didn't sound totally natural, like his hearing when he was younger. But it was a hell of a lot better than wearing both aids. And it was much, much better than going without altogether.

Hearing testing had shown no difference, literally none, between

Ralph's ears in hearing acuity or ability to understand speech. Testing with the aids in place showed that the degree of benefit from both aids was precisely the same. Electro-acoustic analysis of the aids' perform- ance showed that both aids were identical in output, distortion levels, and every other parameter. Conventional theory stated that two ears are always better than one—the listening benefits of binaural hearing have been documented and backed up with years and years of re- search.

Why then, did Ralph have such success with just one aid?

At this point, I was brought into the case. Although I am an audiol- ogist, I no longer dispense hearing aids myself and haven't done so for a long time. My areas of specialty are primarily in diagnostic and man- agement techniques particularly relating to auditory neuroscience, in- cluding APD. Differences between ears or between hearing aids could not account for Ralph's preference for right-ear amplification, so we had to look for more central, brain-related causes.

Further testing revealed that Ralph exhibited a significant deficit in interhemispheric auditory processing. His difficulty was much more pronounced than that of most adults his age. In short, when different information was given to Ralph's right ear than to his left at the same time, the information presented to his right ear had a straight shot to the left side of his brain where speech-sound processing takes place. Information presented to his left ear, however, had to travel first to the right hemisphere. Then it had to cross to the other side before arriving at its final destination. Because Ralph's interhemispheric processing skills were extremely poor, his left ear was at a definite dis- advantage. It is not clear whether the left-ear input arrived later or was distorted, but one thing was certain: Ralph heard far better with just the right ear alone than with the left ear or with both ears in com- bination.

For some elderly people, one hearing aid may actually be more ben- eficial than two. This was certainly the case with Ralph, and with Eve- lyn, from chapter 1. In fact, interhemispheric processing problems are common among elderly listeners and may occur, in some people, as a part of normal aging.

For most people, however, two ears really are better than one. That's why audiologists continue to recommend that binaural hearing aids be tried first. But when a person has a lot of difficulty listening with two hearing aids, it may be useful to try just one aid at a time to see if that improves the situation.

An elderly man or woman may reject hearing aids for many reasons other than interhemispheric processing problems. One may be the stigma attached to hearing aid use—a stigma that, hopefully, is decreasing. Other reasons are behavioral or psychological, such as denial, depression, or a feeling of futility. Still another may be the nature of the individual person's hearing loss—simply put, some hearing losses respond better to amplification than others. Finally, some elderly people experience a condition known as *phonemic regression,* which is extremely poor speech understanding even in quiet environments. This occurs because of significant distortion in the auditory system, and although input is louder with amplification, distortion persists and limits the ability to understand speech at all. All of the listening difficulties experienced by the elderly cannot and should not be attributed to APD, nor should the presence of APD be assumed merely on the basis of someone's age.

APD in the elderly may certainly contribute to hearing difficulties that are present and may make management of hearing loss more difficult. It is important to consider the whole system—from the ear to the brain—when addressing listening problems.

Adults with APD usually find it to be most disruptive at work or at home when oral communication is required. Socially, adults with APD may begin to avoid situations in which they know they will have difficulty—such as cocktail parties, church socials, and the like. Furthermore, listening problems in the elderly are usually attributed to hearing loss alone. Elderly adults with APD may experience even more frustration when hearing aids have limited success in improving

their hearing. Adults with APD may be accused of not paying attention and may be criticized or penalized for their inability to understand or follow through on instructions or verbally presented
information. Their auditory difficulties can lead to significant problems at work, in social situations, and on the home front. In its own
way, APD can be as devastating for the adult as it is for the child.

5

DIAGNOSING APD

I CAN'T COUNT THE number of communications I have received from people—either parents of children with learning problems or people with listening difficulties themselves—who are absolutely certain that they have an APD even before they speak to me. They have gathered snippets of information about the disorder from a variety of sources—other people affected by APD, on-line chat groups, Internet lists of "key indicators," and the available literature—and are convinced that this is the answer they have been seeking for years. Sometimes they have even arrived at a "diagnosis" of APD with the guidance of well-meaning (but misinformed) professionals who are themselves relying on such checklists and communications.

It may not be clear why such rushes to judgment can be dangerous. After all, what can possibly be the harm in assuming that a person has an APD on the basis of limited information, especially if such an assumption leads to therapy techniques that may prove effective? But an accurate diagnosis is absolutely critical in determining how an individual person is affected by APD and in making appropriate, individually designed recommendations for managing the disorder.

WHY YOU NEED TO BE TESTED FOR APD

Not all listening problems are due to APD, although APD certainly does affect a person's ability to listen. Likewise, while APD may cause or be associated with reading, spelling, speech, language, learning, and other difficulties, not all learning and related difficulties are related to APD. To make matters more confusing, many other types of disorders can either coexist with or mimic APD. Attention-deficit/hyperactivity disorder, for example, will certainly affect a person's ability to listen, especially in noisy or distracting environments. Mental retardation, even if very mild, will probably affect a person's ability to process and understand auditory information. Even disorders such as autism can affect language processing and manifest themselves in some ways quite similarly to APD. Yet the treatment for each of these disorders will be very different from those for children or adults with APD. Obtaining a correct diagnosis is the first step in determining what the appropriate treatment should be.

There is an even more important reason why an accurate diagnosis of APD is essential: Not all types of APD are treated in the same manner. If a child or adult does have an APD, the therapy will depend on the specific characteristics of that person's auditory disorder. Depending on the type of APD, some suggestions might actually exacerbate the problem, leading to even greater difficulty at school or work. Even seemingly innocuous management or therapy suggestions can actually be harmful for some types of APD. At the very least, when treatment techniques are applied inappropriately to certain types of APD, valuable time will be wasted, time that could have been spent on appropriate interventions. Accurate diagnosis is critical because it is the only way that appropriate intervention programs can be designed.

HERE'S WHAT YOU NEED TO DO

If some type of hearing or listening problem is suspected, including APD, the first step should be to get a comprehensive hearing test—or audiologic evaluation—performed by an audiologist. If you are the parent of a preschool or school-aged child with such a problem, your best resource will probably be your local school district. Most school districts employ or contract with audiologists with educational and pediatric expertise. Alternatively, you may wish to contact your physician for a referral to an audiologist trained in assessing young children. Adults who suspect some form of hearing or listening problem should also have their hearing tested prior to consideration of a central auditory diagnostic evaluation. A referral by a physician is not necessary for an audiologist to assess hearing, but it may be required by your insurance company for reimbursement purposes. If this is the case, you should contact your doctor for a referral and obtain pre-authorization for the testing from your insurance carrier. For information regarding audiologists in your area, you may wish to contact the American Speech-Language-Hearing Association (1-800-638-8255 or www.asha.org) or the American Academy of Audiology (1-800-AAA-2336 or www.audiology.org). Remember that it is important to consult with an audiologist with pediatric expertise for children suspected of hearing or listening problems. Finally, although hearing screenings may be performed by school nurses, speech-language pathologists, physician's assistants, and a variety of other health-related personnel, a comprehensive hearing evaluation can only be performed by an audiologist.

Once a hearing loss has been ruled out as the primary cause of listening problems, you can discuss your APD concerns with the audiologist. If you are an adult, the audiologist may recommend central auditory testing based on your history and symptoms. But if you are the parent of a child suspected of APD, the audiologist will probably want to make sure that tests of language, cognition, and related abilities have been completed first to explore the child's overall functioning. APD is merely one, small possible factor contributing to language and learning problems in children. It should never be a starting point in the diagnostic process. We will discuss later how the results of a child's tests are used both to indicate the need for central auditory testing and to help us determine how an APD may be affecting a child in his or her daily life. For now, though, it is important to understand that these assessments should be completed prior to any evaluations for possible APD.

If your child is having difficulties in school, these tests may already have been completed as part of an educational evaluation to determine eligibility for special education services. If they have not been completed, you should speak with your child's teacher or other educational professional about obtaining these assessments through the school district. If the educational team does not feel that such testing is indicated for your child, you may need to pursue these assessments on your own through local speech-language pathologists, psychologists, and other professionals. Your physician, local or state university, or audiologist can help you find resources in your area for these types of tests.

When all of the information is in place, a decision will be made whether a central auditory evaluation for APD is necessary. At that time, you will be referred to an audiologist trained in APD evaluation. This audiologist may be employed by the school district or a local university speech and hearing clinic or may be in private practice. Not all audiologists are trained in APD diagnosis, so it is important to find one with the necessary expertise. Once again, if your health insurance requires pre-authorization for reimbursement purposes, you will probably need to obtain a physician's referral for this testing prior to making an appointment. Some insurance companies do not reimburse for APD testing, so you should discuss this with your health insurance provider. If your child's educational team has decided that the testing is necessary, however, they will probably pay for the APD assessment or provide it free of charge to your child.

Finally, I should emphasize that not everyone can be tested for APD. A child must be at least seven or eight years of age before a behavioral central auditory evaluation can be completed, although some types of brain-wave, or electrophysiologic, testing can be completed at much younger ages that will give some idea of the functioning of the central auditory nervous system. A hearing loss may interfere with the ability to assess central auditory function. Significant cognitive, language, or related difficulties such as those that occur with mental retardation, autism, AD/HD, or other disorders may indicate that an

APD evaluation is not necessary or cannot be performed. All these factors will be taken into account when deciding whether a central auditory assessment can or should be completed.

THE DIAGNOSTIC JOURNEY: HERE'S WHAT WILL HAPPEN

Because a central auditory evaluation requires a good deal of attention and effort, I usually try to schedule young children for APD assessment in the morning when they are less likely to be fatigued and can put forth their best effort. Other audiologists may perform these evaluations throughout the day. The entire assessment may take as long as three hours, so it is important that we test children when they are best able to listen and attend.

When you arrive for your (or your child's) appointment, the audiologist will probably begin with a detailed interview, especially if he or she has not met you previously. This interview will consist of a variety of questions designed to explore the types of difficulties you or your child is having in various situations. You may also be asked to fill out questionnaires regarding listening and related behaviors. The audiologist should be familiar with your particular situation by reviewing the results of previous educational, speech-language, and cognitive test results prior to your appointment. Nevertheless, your subjective impressions, symptoms, and complaints should be taken into account. At this time, it is critical to share all information openly with the audiologist. I have found that some parents may wish to hide information that is uncomfortable for them for fear that the audiologist will be negatively influenced (for example, previous diagnoses with which the parents disagree—autism, mental retardation, AD/HD—or test results that they feel are inaccurate or unreliable). However, parents must understand that an accurate diagnosis of APD and the development of an appropriate management plan can only occur if all information is discussed and taken into account. The audiologist's job is to remain objective while, at the same time, considering all of the evidence available in arriving at a diagnosis.

For the central auditory testing itself, you (or your child) will be placed in a sound-shielded test booth and headphones will be used. Several tests will be performed that may include listening to words, tones, numbers, sentences, and other auditory signals and reporting what was heard in a variety of ways. If fatigue or lack of attention becomes a concern, breaks may be provided, especially when testing young children or people with attention disorders. In my practice, I rarely have the parents present during testing because I have found that most children pay attention and perform better when it is just the two of us. Other audiologists may include parents. The actual testing may take as little as forty-five minutes or as long as two hours, depending on the person being tested and the tests that are chosen.

When the testing is completed, the results may be shared at that time or later. I usually interpret and provide counseling regarding the results immediately following the completion of the assessment. Sometimes, however, detailed analysis is needed before the results of an evaluation can be shared. In any case, the results of the assessment should indicate whether an APD is present, the characteristics of the APD, and how the APD relates to the person's listening, learning, and communication complaints. Finally, when the results of the central auditory evaluation are considered together with the previous educational and related information, specific recommendations for management and treatment should be an integral part of the diagnostic report.

This has been just a brief overview of what typically occurs during a central auditory assessment. Following is a more detailed discussion of central auditory test procedures.

TOOLS OF THE TRADE:
DIAGNOSTIC TESTS FOR APD

APD can be formally diagnosed only by an audiologist because of the nature of the test tools used in an APD diagnosis. These tools require excellent acoustic control and all of the machinery, bells, and whistles that are a part of the audiologist's practice, including sound booths, audiometers, signal delivery systems, and electrophysiologic equipment. Because of the need for this specialized equipment, along with specific training in auditory-based deficits, the audiologist is the designated professional to diagnose APD.

However, not all audiologists are trained in central auditory diagnosis and treatment. In fact, it might be said that many, even most, are not. But awareness of and education in this important field are increasing daily. Until recently, APD either was not covered in many of our educational programs, or was touched on only lightly, providing insufficient information for a clinician to actually put his or her knowledge into practice. APD requires knowledge in many professional areas. An audiologist needs to know about cognition, language, learning, and related topics to be truly proficient at assessing and managing APD. Obtaining this training and education can be challenging for many clinicians who are already "in the trenches" because they must actively seek out continuing-education activities, including "shadowing" other clinicians, attending workshops, and taking additional college courses.

Furthermore, our field has evolved in many ways into specialty areas. All audiologists are trained to assess a person's hearing sensitivity and related capabilities. Some audiologists dispense hearing aids, others do not. Some audiologists work primarily in adult settings, such as clinics or hospitals. Others focus primarily on pediatric audiology, including working in the schools or in clinics or hospitals that see a good number of children. Some audiologists are trained in (and have available to them equipment for) the full complement of electrophysiologic measures. Others may focus primarily on brain-stem function alone or not perform any electrophysiologic testing at all. Although most of us have a smattering of experience and training running the full gamut of audiology, what tends to happen is that the audiologist's practice setting and personal interests ultimately determine those areas in which he or she becomes most proficient. Although we may be able to take on other roles in a pinch, we may be far from truly competent in those areas.

Audiologists who work in certain adult-focused hospital or clinical settings may not have a lot of experience testing the hearing of very young children—a task that requires special knowledge and skills. If a small child needs a hearing test, we recommend that this be pursued with a clinician who has experience and expertise in pediatric audiology.

School-based audiologists may seem the obvious choice to have experience with APD. However, we need to remember the incredible caseloads many of these clinicians are struggling under. Many areas have only one audiologist for several districts, and that audiologist is responsible for screening, testing, monitoring amplification, and a variety of other duties for all of the children in the locale. This may leave little time for a school-based audiologist to undergo training and engage in the time-consuming assessment and management of APD. We should never assume that all audiologists provide services related to APD any more than we should assume that all cardiac surgeons are proficient at heart transplantation.

How, then, can you find an audiologist who has expertise in APD and provides assessment and management of auditory-based processing deficits? First of all, ask. Your local school district, speech-language pathologist, physician, psychologist, or tutor may know of someone in your area who provides these services. However, I should emphasize that APD services simply are not available in many areas of this country and abroad. You may need to travel to obtain a central auditory evaluation.

To obtain information regarding audiologists who provide central auditory processing services, you may contact your state's Speech-Language-Hearing Association or Academy of Audiology. Our national audiologists' governing organizations also keep databases of such referral information. Finally, the recent appearance of an Internet-based support and information resource for people interested in auditory processing disorders—the National Coalition for Auditory Processing Disorders, Inc. (NCAPD)—has made finding a professional who specializes in APD easier than ever. They can be accessed at www.ncapd.org.

Once you have found an audiologist who can provide central auditory assessment services, what should you expect from such an assessment and how do you know if you have received quality services? The following is a general guide of what should be expected from such an evaluation:

1. The audiologist should take a complete case history, including questions regarding the types of difficulties the person is having, specific learning, language, communication, and cognitive concerns, and developmental, family, and medical topics.

2. The audiologist should be familiar with the results of previous tests of language, learning, communication, and cognition. Although I require that these records be available to me prior to consideration for a central auditory evaluation, some audiologists may not do so. However, it is important that the audiologist not attempt to diagnose APD in a vacuum, and that the testing and results, as well as recommendations for management, be directed toward the person's individual areas of difficulty and pattern of complaints.

3. The testing should be conducted in a sound-shielded booth using audiologic equipment. A variety of auditory processes should be addressed, including dichotic listening (listening to a different signal in each ear simultaneously), perception of dis-

torted speech (which may consist of filtered speech or very rapid, time-compressed speech, among others), perception of nonverbal auditory stimuli (including tone patterns), temporal (or time-based) auditory processing, and perhaps others. The actual names of the tests may vary; however, tests that are referred to as "screening" tools or that are not administered in a sound booth (such as many speech and language auditory perceptual measures or psychological tests) should not be considered diagnostic tests for APD, although they may provide valuable information about the person's overall listening or comprehension abilities.

4. The audiologist should spend sufficient time explaining the tests used and the results of such tests. In my practice, I often describe test results in terms of *left-hemisphere, right-hemisphere,* and *interhemispheric abilities* to help the patients and their families understand the nature of the test tools used and what the results mean. Although there are several different theoretical models of APD, the important point is that the patient and family understand what was done and how the patient performed on each test.

5. If the results indicate that the person does, indeed, exhibit an auditory processing deficit, the nature of the deficit and how it relates to the person's language, learning, and communication difficulties should be described in terms understandable to the layperson. Just as it is critical not to diagnose APD in a vacuum, it is critical that the results of central auditory testing not be interpreted in a vacuum. That is, the outcome of a central auditory assessment should not be just the identification of an APD—a yes-or-no response. Instead, the results should be used to define the disorder and determine how that disorder contributes to the person's functional difficulties.

6. Finally, when an APD is confirmed, the results of the evaluation, when taken together with all of the other information about the

child or the adult, should result in specific suggestions for management. These suggestions may include ways to manage the listening environment, methods of compensating for the disorder, and specific therapy techniques. Management should be individualized. In other words, the treatment should apply directly to the individual person's patterns of difficulty and auditory-based deficit. You should get more for your money than merely a preprinted laundry list of suggestions "helpful for people with APD." Appropriate management strategies vary depending on the nature of the APD. Therefore, if the only outcome of a diagnostic central auditory evaluation is the confirmation of the presence of APD and the handing over of a general list of suggestions that is not individualized and provides no specific directions for intervention, you might just as well have requested a copy of the handout in the first place and not bothered with the evaluation at all.

Other things you should expect from any comprehensive central auditory assessment are ample time for the patient and/or family to ask questions, willingness of the audiologist to be a team player and to communicate with educational service providers or others engaged in the management of the person's difficulties, and a written report delineating all of the information outlined above. In addition, if recommendations for additional evaluations are made, such as medical follow-up, electrophysiologic measures, neuropsychologic consult, and the like, the rationale underlying such recommendations should be explained clearly.

Finally, the topic of who pays for a central auditory evaluation should be addressed. Many parents of children suspected of APD expect their school district either to provide such services or to pay for an assessment by an outside audiologist. The school district may pay for such testing, but only if the multidisciplinary educational team has determined that this evaluation is necessary for educational purposes and has formally recommended it. When this is not the case, typically the family must pay for a private evaluation. At present, some health insurers will cover an APD evaluation, while others will not. Many audiologists will not file insurance for the patient, but will instead require payment up front and will provide the family with documentation so that they can file the necessary papers themselves. Often, if a family is unable to afford these services, financial assistance through service organizations or through the clinic itself may be available.

THE LANGUAGE, LEARNING, AND COMMUNICATION PUZZLE

To avoid the possibility of different, often contrasting, diagnoses and recommendations for management, it is critical that specialists not operate in a vacuum. First and foremost, the entire person should be taken into account. Although I have already emphasized the need for multidisciplinary collaboration, it certainly bears mentioning once again. We must take a holistic approach to the diagnosis of APD, or any related language, learning, or communication disorder. If auditory processing is focused on exclusively, we can be led down the wrong path entirely. Consideration of and testing for APD should *never* be a starting point in the diagnostic process.

Ultimately, however, we do need to analyze the nature of those areas in which the person has difficulties. In particular, we want to look for patterns that suggest that certain brain regions are not functioning properly. We also want to look for patterns that are consistent with APD. In some situations, our analysis will indicate that a primary APD is not the likely culprit in the person's difficulties, after all. Instead, the analysis may suggest that other, nonauditory disorders and avenues should be explored. In other situations, valuable information about how a possible APD may be affecting a person's specific skill areas will guide us in the direction our treatment efforts should take.

In my own practice, I do not see children for APD assessment until they have had some form of assessment of overall language, cognition, and academic abilities, as well as any other areas of concern. There is a simple reason for this. Auditory processing is merely one small, albeit important, piece in the larger language, learning, and communication puzzle. Without information on the other pieces of the puzzle, specific information that clearly delineates the child's difficulties, I cannot even begin to determine whether my own test results are consistent with the other information. I also cannot design a management program that will be meaningful to that particular child.

It simply makes no sense to jump to a hypothesis of APD in a child with language or communication difficulties. An assessment by a speech-language pathologist, the professional uniquely qualified to address language disorders, would be the logical, appropriate first step. I have seen many cases in which children have exhibited language concerns even from infancy or toddlerhood, yet have never seen a language specialist. Instead, they have been evaluated by a variety of other specialists. You wouldn't consult an orthopedist for a sore throat.

Concerns about learning and academic achievement beg for an assessment of the child's learning and achievement—usually by a psychologist or educational diagnostician. Similarly, any time processing of information is a concern, a look at the child's overall cognitive processing abilities is in order—which requires the services of a psychologist or psychiatrist trained in such assessment. Always keep in mind individual professionals' scopes of practice. A psychologist or psychiatrist alone cannot diagnose language disorders. A speech-language pathologist alone cannot diagnose psychological or cognitive disorders. A pediatrician or primary-care physician alone cannot diagnose either type of disorder. And none of them can diagnose APD. Therefore, a team approach is crucial to arrive at a consensus of diagnosis (or set of diagnoses) in any given case.

So first we begin with those assessments that will evaluate, in depth, the person's presenting difficulties. In most cases involving APD, especially in children, these presenting difficulties cross language, academic/learning, and cognitive domains, requiring assessments of these areas before the possible presence of a specific auditory-based deficit can be addressed. Think of it as a "systems check," just as would be done with any type of physical illness, the same type of systems check that is undertaken when trying to troubleshoot why a computer program is crashing all the time or why our car is not working properly.

ASSESSING THE WHOLE PERSON

We should begin the diagnostic journey with a look at the person in his or her entirety to gain a picture of strengths and weaknesses across domains. All too often, we focus on what the child or adult *can't* do. But it is equally important, if not more so, to focus on what the person *can* do. An individual's strengths are important both as a part of the diagnostic picture and to provide a stable starting point from which he or she can begin to grow. This is known as a holistic approach to diagnosis. The other alternative, known as the disability model of assessing and treating disorder, focuses specifically on the deficit area. This approach is not only disheartening for all involved, but it often fails to take into account the interrelationship between the disorder and the person's quality of life and performance in other areas. From the overall picture of the person's ease or difficulty across a variety of skills, we will determine whether APD may be a likely suspect in his or her difficulties.

I always ask children what their favorite subject in school is, and what their least favorite is. I then probe to find out why they have identified those particular subjects: Is it because those areas are particularly easy or difficult for them, or is it due to other factors (boredom with the subject matter or dislike for a strict teacher)?

I once met a young girl in the fourth grade, Kara, who said reading was her absolute favorite class and math her absolute least favorite. Yet Kara had been referred to me, at least in part, because of severe difficulties in reading and spelling, which had led me to expect that she would identify reading as a problem area. But when Kara spoke of her reading teacher, her eyes took on a shine that can only be described as love. Her reading resource teacher, with whom she had been working for two years, was a lovely young woman who was kind and patient and supportive—all of the qualities kids respond to in a teacher. She had never made Kara feel inadequate for her reading or spelling difficulties; rather, she had spent a good deal of time assisting Kara with her assignments and always applauded even the smallest of successes. As a result, Kara had not yet experienced the spiral into disillusionment and subsequent hate/avoidance of reading that often accompanies reading and spelling disorders. She looked forward every day to working in this most frustrating area because this one woman had motivated her so strongly. Of course, once we reached the management stage with Kara, her reading resource teacher was heavily involved in the implementation, which assured some degree of success right at the outset—one example of why it is important to consider all aspects of the child's life when undertaking diagnosis and management of APD.

On the other hand, Kara hated math. When questioned, however, we discovered that math was easy, too easy, for her. Indeed, she usually completed her math worksheets entirely accurately in less than half of the time allotted, while the rest of the students in the class usually required the entire period. And in that particular class, if students completed their worksheets early, they were instructed to use their "free" time by—you guessed it—reading. Without the support of her reading resource teacher, Kara struggled with independent reading. What many of us dream of—free time just to read for pleasure—was perceived by Kara almost as a punishment for getting her work done early and performing it well. Thus, our questions helped to illuminate how Kara's most difficult subject could be her favorite and her easiest subject could be her least favorite, as well as giving us some ideas right away for a few classroom-based management suggestions.

In adults also, identifying the areas in which they experience the most frustration and those in which they excel is important for subsequent management, as well as for determining the ways in which a disorder may be affecting their quality of life. It also tells us who might need to be involved in management/intervention. For example, the corporate executive who reports little difficulty in the office but extreme difficulty communicating with his wife and four children will probably have little interest in or need for information regarding the Americans with Disabilities Act (ADA) or for methods of coping with a disorder in the workplace. However, it may become critical to involve his family in the diagnostic process right from the outset, and to focus on including them in the counseling so that they are better able to understand his communication difficulties. It may also be useful to have the family members themselves come up with ways to improve communication in the home so that suggestions and strategies will more likely be implemented.

Nothing can take the place of direct observation of a child or an adult in his or her daily environment. Sometimes we can identify environmental factors that exacerbate any type of learning, language, or communication difficulty, such as excess noise spilling over from a nearby classroom. Sometimes, these environmental factors may not be apparent to the teachers and students who are in the room every day. For example, they may have become accustomed to and ignore the buzz of a fluorescent lightbulb. Yet, that persistent buzz will probably affect everyone's ability to hear in that classroom. Therefore, an observer new to the environment can often provide a fresh perspective and identify possible problems.

The environment is not the only thing that should be carefully observed. The behavior of the person in that environment should be an equal, if not more important, object of our focus. Sometimes, our observations confirm the descriptions we've been given. Sometimes, however, our observations do not jibe with the information that has been provided by parents, teachers, or concerned others.

The most striking example in my own career was a third-grade girl

who was having difficulty understanding and following verbally presented directions in the classroom, along with a variety of academic
problems. Questionnaires filled out by her teachers and parents indicated that Lexy, when compared to same-age peers in the classroom
and to her own siblings, seemed able to sustain attention well, was cooperative and tried hard, yet had difficulty with a variety of tasks
across many domains. She was in danger of being held back at the end
of the school year. But in one-on-one testing sessions, Lexy was
friendly, cooperative, and appeared to have little difficulty completing
the tasks required of her. Indeed, Lexy performed pretty well on all
standardized tests of cognitive, academic, and language functioning,
although she did occasionally have to be redirected when her attention
seemed to wander. She also had to be told to sit still at times when she
began to bounce her leg up and down or wiggle in her chair.

When I observed Lexy in the classroom, I was surprised by what I
saw. Contrary to reports, I found that Lexy remained on task less than
5 percent of the time. She spent virtually all of her energy on other activities: playing with a pencil set or worrying a frayed shoelace on her
boot, counting the tiles in the ceiling or doodling on her desk. She
rarely looked at the teacher when she was speaking. Other times Lexy
would stare out the window dreamily, with a faraway expression on
her face that clearly showed that she *was not there.* Even when she was
watching the teacher, Lexy often had this blank look on her face.
When asked a direct question, she would subtly shake her head as if
physically dragging herself back into the present, only to be unable to
answer accurately.

Why, you might ask, did the teacher not see these behaviors as
clearly as I, an outside observer, saw them? Once again, observation of
the class provided the answer. The teacher-to-student ratio in that
urban classroom was one to twenty-eight. And of those twenty-eight
students, three had been diagnosed with AD/HD. These three boys
seemed to spend more time out of their seats than in them, distracting
everyone and requiring constant reinstruction and refocusing. Invari-

ably, once one of the boys settled down, another jumped up, and so on, a vicious cycle that repeated again and again so that, by the end of the day, the teacher seemed literally exhausted from trying to keep these three boys on task and still provide ample attention to the remaining twenty-five students.

Throughout all of this, there sat Lexy, in comparison quiet, attentive, never making a scene or distracting others, well-behaved, compliant. Only when she was the sole focus of observation over a long period—a luxury that I had but that the teacher did not—did her own inattentiveness become apparent.

A similar situation was found at home. Lexy was the oldest of five siblings, and her home was chaotic and noisy with five kids and two dogs running around. In contrast to her active and playful younger brothers and sisters, Lexy would come home at the end of the day and sit quietly watching television or playing computer games. Indeed, as her parents had stated, she did seem to have an excellent ability to sustain attention—almost too excellent. Lexy exhibited the ability to *hyperfocus,* to become completely absorbed in one thing to the absolute exclusion of everything else for long periods, a behavior that is common to many attention deficits but that is often overlooked. Many people do not realize that AD/HD does not always consist of hyperactivity or the complete inability to pay attention, but sometimes, may also include the ability to pay attention *far too well,* as was the case with Lexy at times.

Ultimately, Lexy was indeed diagnosed with AD/HD, inattentive type with no associated hyperactivity. Her ability to pay attention in one-on-one situations, such as during standardized testing, was not uncommon, as many children with this disorder do quite well under focused attention. Subsequent medical intervention proved effective with Lexy, and we ended up never contemplating a central auditory diagnosis at all.

Lexy's case illustrates how important it is to step back and look at the whole person and his or her functioning in real-life, daily environments. When we focus on one small part or ability—such as auditory processing—and do so in an artificial, one-on-one testing situation, many insights into the person's overall functioning and other areas of strength or weakness may be entirely obscured. As a result, we may take an entirely wrong path on our diagnostic journey.

Although we should always try to identify areas of difficulty that affect daily functioning, it is equally important to focus on those areas that the person enjoys or excels at. Identifying a person's areas of strength assists in developing or maintaining self-esteem and feelings of self-worth and success. It can also provide critical information about which areas of the brain are functioning properly. For example, the child with good math calculation abilities and visual-spatial skills, who is good at music and art and can put blocks together to form a desired object and see the overall pattern in problem-solving activities or puzzles, probably exhibits intact right-hemisphere abilities. This information allows us to begin narrowing our search for the specific type or areas of dysfunction the person is experiencing and to rule out higher-order cognitive deficits that affect functioning across all domains. In this way, we can make preliminary predictions regarding possible difficulty areas that may arise so that they may be headed off before they become a significant problem.

This information also provides us with a starting point for many of our therapy and intervention activities. Perhaps art abilities will come in handy during note-taking or listening to directions. Perhaps visualization abilities can also be relied upon. Maybe therapy involving speech sounds or words set to music will be more appropriate for the person who excels at music. Whatever we can do to make therapy and management more enjoyable will increase the likelihood that our suggestions will be complied with and therapy will be successful.

DISASSEMBLY REQUIRED: ANALYZING AREAS OF WEAKNESS

Our next step is to determine whether an APD evaluation is indicated. In my approach, particularly when working with school-aged children, I try to answer four key questions, using the information supplied by the assessments of language, learning, cognition, and other areas:

1. Are the current evaluations sufficient in scope to begin consideration of possible APD?

2. Do the results of the current evaluations suggest the likelihood of an APD, or might this person's difficulties be due to other factors?

3. Can the person participate in an auditory processing evaluation?

4. Will the results of an APD evaluation add anything to the current management plan?

1. Are the current evaluations sufficient in scope to begin consideration of possible APD? Information from a variety of skill areas should be obtained prior to jumping to the conclusion that someone has an APD. For an adult suspected of APD, a complete audiologic (hearing) assessment may be sufficient. However, if the adult has suffered a recent stroke or head trauma or is returning to college and experiencing learning difficulties, more comprehensive evaluations of language, learning, and cognition may be necessary.

For children, thorough evaluations of primary areas of difficulties are usually required before I will begin assessment of central auditory function. Thus, if the child has language difficulties, a language evaluation is necessary. If there are learning concerns, a cognitive and learning evaluation is needed. If AD/HD is suspected, this should be either diagnosed or ruled out prior to APD assessment. Although AD/HD and APD can coexist, they also can mimic one another. If medical interventions are required for AD/HD (for example, the use of Ritalin or a similar medication), these should be in place prior to central auditory testing because it will help to remove attention-related confounds that may affect my test results. Other general issues such as overall health and possible seizure or neurological disorders should also be investigated prior to focusing on the one, small piece of the puzzle that is auditory processing.

2. Do the results of the current evaluations suggest the likelihood of an APD, or might this person's difficulties be due to other factors? This is one of the most important questions, and it can only be answered through a multidisciplinary team approach that takes into account the findings of all previous evaluations, observations, and history. We are looking for specific patterns that suggest that the person's difficulties may be due to auditory-based, "bottom-up" or input processing factors rather than higher-order cognitive, linguistic, attention, or other factors. All of the information discussed in the previous chapters of this book is taken into account when attempting to answer question two.

For example, reading requires everything from basic sound-symbol association and visual perception to cognitive processes such as memory and inferential thinking. When a child has reading difficulties, we comb the records carefully and look for difficulties in specific areas important for reading. The child who exhibits poor visual-processing and scanning abilities, has difficulty visually distinguishing one letter from another, cannot identify numbers along with letters, and seems to respond well to visual interventions such as colored filters on the page or rulers to assist line scanning is probably not a child with APD. This is particularly true if the child does better with verbally presented information. The child who exhibits good phonological word-attack and sight-word abilities, discriminates easily among similar-sounding words or speech sounds, reads rapidly or with high accuracy, but has difficulty comprehending or remembering what is read is probably experiencing a higher-level language, cognitive, or memory disorder and not an APD. This is especially true if the child also has difficulty remembering or understanding directions or information, especially when complex, yet can hear and repeat (and even comprehend) the directions or information at the time of presentation—although some children with APD do display difficulty in this latter area.

On the other hand, the child who exhibits poor phonological awareness abilities and mishears similar-sounding words or speech sounds, which then *leads to* slow reading and lack of comprehension of what is read may well be exhibiting a primary APD affecting reading. Likewise, the child with poor sight word abilities, combined with other right-hemisphere findings such as math calculation difficulties, social language concerns, difficulty comprehending tone-of-voice cues, and visual-spatial problems, may require central auditory assessment to determine whether right-hemisphere-based auditory processing abilities are affected.

As a general rule, when we see evidence that a child exhibits difficulty across most or all areas, regardless of the area of the brain on which the skills rely or the type of processing abilities required, we begin to suspect something "larger than" APD—something more global and involving higher-level cognitive function. Similarly, when behaviors or difficulties cannot reasonably be attributed to or connected with auditory-based deficit, such as self-stimulating behaviors (hand-flapping, rocking), lack of eye contact, persistent or occasional inability to distinguish between fantasy and reality, frequent episodes of spacing out with a blank look, and so on, we must consider the possibility of a neurological or other higher-order disorder. Certainly, any disorder of language, cognition, attention, or any other brain function can have an adverse affect on a child's ability to "listen," but that is not the same as saying that the child has an auditory processing deficit.

Moreover, many tests of "auditory perception" or "auditory processing" that are included in psychological or language evaluations actually
assess the ability to listen and involve abilities that are not truly
auditory-specific. Although they may provide valuable information regarding the child's listening or language processing abilities, they are
impacted by higher-order language, cognitive, attention, or other confounds. Because of this, these types of tests should be considered
screening tools only and should never be used to diagnose APD.

When reviewing areas of weakness and analyzing results of prior
evaluations, we must take into account the particular behaviors and
skills required by each subtest of each evaluation. Using the patterns
we find in this information, we must determine whether an auditory-
based deficit can reasonably be a primary contributing factor to the
overall difficulties exhibited by the child.

For adults, this process is usually somewhat less involved. For many
adults, the primary question to be answered is, does he or she experience listening difficulties that are out of proportion to, or cannot be
reasonably attributed to, peripheral hearing loss?

3. Can the person participate in an auditory processing evaluation?
For the most part, behavioral tests of central auditory processing require a mental age of about seven or eight before they can be administered reliably. This is because the rate of maturation of the brain varies
so widely in children six years and younger. For most of our best tests
of central auditory function, anything from 0 to 100 percent may be
within normal limits for very young children, rendering us unable to
interpret our test results even if we can get the child to participate in
the testing. Although elecrophysiologic measures may provide some
information regarding brain function, these tests only provide information on how well the nerves in the central auditory nervous system
fire in synchrony. Not all APD results in asynchrony of neural firing,
and many cases may thus go undetected by electrophysiologic testing.

Our options are truly limited when it comes to testing very young children who are suspected of APD. In these cases, we often rely on a best-guess hypothesis as to the presence and possible nature(s) of an APD. This hypothesis is based on all of the presenting evidence from evaluations, electrophysiologic assessment (when undertaken), and behavioral observation. We then design a management plan based on that hypothesis. In this way, we can address the most likely auditory difficulties at an early age when brain plasticity is at its best. We must realize, however, that an actual APD often cannot be definitively diagnosed until the child is older.

When I receive a communication from a parent or other professional in which a child has been "diagnosed" with APD at age two or three, I always view this information with a good deal of suspicion. Given our current test measures, it is highly unlikely that an actual diagnosis could have been made at so young an age. Furthermore, I frequently find that the terms *language processing* and *auditory processing* are used interchangeably by many professionals both within and outside of my field. Thus, potentially any difficulty with understanding language—spoken or written—can be tagged with the currently popular label APD. Although it is difficult, if not impossible, to draw a distinct line between where audition leaves off and language begins, this does not mean that the two terms are completely interchangeable. In most cases, I am much more comfortable acknowledging a "language processing disorder" in a young child who clearly exhibits difficulties understanding language as opposed to automatically assuming an underlying APD right from the outset. In any case, what is most important is to direct intervention toward the child's key behavioral difficulties.

Many reasons other than age may prevent a person from participating in an auditory processing evaluation. One key consideration is whether he or she has sufficient cognitive capacity to do so. Although some professionals require normal cognitive abilities (or a normal IQ) before they will administer a central auditory evaluation, my own requirements are not quite so strict. For me, the bottom line is whether the person can reliably complete the tasks required. Therefore, if someone is unable to repeat sentences in isolation, he will probably not be able to repeat similar sentences presented in a competing (or dichotic) condition. Similarly, if repeating three or four numbers in isolation is a huge challenge, how can I expect numbers to be repeated when presented dichotically? If someone has difficulty with a standard hearing test or with repeating words in quiet, ideal listening conditions, I certainly cannot expect reliable results from more complex auditory tasks involving the repetition of words under distorted listening conditions. Therefore, rather than relying solely on IQ to determine eligibility for central auditory testing, I rely more on descriptions of behaviors and abilities during related evaluations. These descriptions will illuminate the person's ability (or inability) to participate in the required tasks.

Another aspect that should be considered is the listener's ability to sustain attention. We have seen that AD/HD and APD can occur individually or can coexist. An untreated AD/HD can prevent an accurate auditory processing evaluation since that requires the ability to sit and listen for some time. Although we provide frequent breaks and re-instruction if needed, if someone is unable to stay still or to attend for longer than just a few seconds, determining whether deficits uncovered in our auditory testing are due to an auditory disorder or to the inability to attend to the task will be difficult if not impossible. For this reason, I require anyone suspected of AD/HD to be evaluated and, if indicated, treated for it before consideration of central auditory testing.

Hearing sensitivity is another area that can affect our ability to test for suspected APD. To be interpreted accurately, most of our behavioral tests rely on normal—or at least symmetrical—hearing sensitivity. Although some behavioral tests of central auditory processing can be administered despite some degree of hearing loss as long as the stimuli can be heard, others do require normal hearing sensitivity. Significant hearing loss, ear disease, unilateral (one-eared) or asymmetrical hearing loss, or other ear-related factors may prevent APD diagnostic testing. Even though APD can coexist with, and exacerbate the adverse effects of, hearing loss, our ability to test children or adults with significant or asymmetrical hearing impairments is as yet limited. Therefore, hearing sensitivity and the general health of the ears must be considered before testing for APD.

4. Will the results of an APD evaluation add anything to the current management plan? We should always ask what we expect to gain from a diagnosis of APD. In most situations, the determination of the presence and nature of an APD leads directly to the development of a specific management program. However, I have come across a few situations in which the current management program for a particular person is so comprehensive—and has included specific auditory-based training that seems appropriate—that I wonder what I might be able to add of value. Especially in those cases in which a child is showing good progress, I always let the parents and other service providers know that, even if a central auditory evaluation is undertaken, their current strategies and interventions are so on target that my input may be of little benefit. In some of these cases, the parents and other professionals choose to defer central auditory assessment until later. On the other hand, there may be valid reasons to pursue such an evaluation even under these circumstances.

Just having an appropriate label and a description of the underlying mechanisms of a disorder can go a long way to promote understanding and acceptance of the disorder, as well as to improve the child's self-image. When considering APD and school-aged children, however, it should be noted that the label APD alone is not now a qualifying condition for special education services in virtually any state in the country. Although in some states the label APD may be included under the special education eligibility condition of "speech-language disorder" or "learning disability," it typically does not stand alone. Therefore, the child must meet his or her particular state's eligibility criteria under accepted labels, such as specific learning disability or speech-language, to obtain special education services through the schools under IDEA legislation. A label of APD—if desired for the purpose of obtaining services through the schools—may be all but useless unless additional special education eligibility criteria are met.

I often see a central auditory evaluation requested, even if I am uncertain how much I may be able to contribute to the intervention plan, because many parents, service providers, or others want verification that they are, indeed, moving in the right direction. A central auditory evaluation, accompanied by deficit-specific recommendations, not only validates their own approach but may also guide them in determining therapeutic priorities and weeding out less necessary interventions.

Not all people considering central auditory evaluation come to the assessment from the school system. Some are adults looking for methods of managing auditory difficulties at home or at work. In addition, I often encounter parents seeking recommendations for their children with communication difficulties, no matter how mild. This may occur even if the difficulties are not affecting the child sufficiently to qualify him or her for special education services. For many of these parents, home-based or private therapy has been successful and has resulted in an improvement in communication or related skills for their child. They are also trying to obtain as much information as possible to make sure that they are exploring every avenue. Some of these children might be eligible for some school-based accommodations under Statute 504 of the Americans with Disabilities Act, which requires a specific diagnosis.

In conclusion, it is important to determine what contribution an APD diagnosis will likely make to the overall management program prior to committing both the time and money for the evaluations required. If a central auditory evaluation is still indicated, for any of the reasons cited above, and if all of the preceding questions have also been answered yes, then it is time to take that next step in the diagnostic journey.

I should emphasize that, if it is determined that a central auditory evaluation is not indicated for any of the above four reasons, that does not mean that the person does not exhibit an APD. Conversely, just because all evidence points strongly toward an APD in a given case, that does not mean that an APD *has been* diagnosed. Only a diagnostic central auditory evaluation can answer these questions.

INTEGRATING TEST RESULTS

Once the diagnostic process has been completed, the pieces of the puzzle should be reassembled so that a management program that addresses that person's issues may be designed. A diagnosis of APD should always lead to a meaningful, well-thought-out, individualized management plan.

When we integrate test results, our primary focus is on the identification of patterns across academic, language, cognitive, and related findings; areas of reported difficulties; and the tests of central auditory function themselves. Because we are testing several different processes and brain areas, we would not expect a child or adult with APD to perform poorly on all central auditory tests. This finding would suggest a more global cognitive or attention-based problem, or that the listener was not putting forth his or her best effort. Although a true APD might be buried in the findings, we can't identify or define it. When poor performance is seen on every single test, the possible auditory piece of the puzzle is most likely not the biggest, most important contributing factor to the person's listening difficulties, anyway.

Several years ago, I assessed a young man who had at a very young age been diagnosed as mentally retarded. I tested this child against my better judgment, and only because his mother had pleaded with me to take a look at her boy. Randy demonstrated an overall IQ of 68—on paper, at least—with equally developed abilities in virtually all cognitive areas. His IQ definitely placed him in the range of mental retardation. Randy had been retested twice since his initial evaluation, and each retest had shown the same results. He had been placed in a self-contained classroom for handicapped students at age six, and because this was many years ago in a low-income, rural area, his education was less than ideal. Randy's classmates were children with many different types and severities of disabilities. For the most part, Randy spent his class time under a table in the corner, looking through picture books. Because he was compliant and friendly, and because some of the other children in the classroom required intensive monitoring and assistance, Randy often went unnoticed.

Randy's mother contacted me after hearing me speak at a local learning-disabilities conference. She said that she had always mistrusted the diagnosis of mental retardation and that she *knew* Randy was brighter than the test results showed. However, because of the lack of services in her area and her own limited income, she had been unable to find anyone to confirm her suspicion. She had forwarded all of Randy's testing to me. His testing clearly documented deficits in all areas time and time again and was consistent with his diagnosis of mental retardation. I could find not even a scintilla of evidence that Randy had been misdiagnosed. Instead, I believed that his mother might still be caught up in the gut-wrenching cycle of denial that often accompanies the diagnosis of a disability in a child. Basically, I knew that this was not a child with APD and therefore, I denied her request for testing and gently tried to explain why I felt my services were inappropriate.

However, she was persistent. She asked me just to talk with Randy. She felt sure I would recognize what was so apparent to her: that, although something certainly was wrong with him, he wasn't mentally retarded. Finally, I agreed to meet with her and her son, just to talk.

I spoke with Randy for only a short time before I began to see what his mother meant. At times, Randy talked about hobbies and school using well-developed language. During these periods, he could understand even relatively complex sentences and questions. But at other times, Randy would merely stare at me blankly, completely unable to comprehend what I was saying. One minute, he could answer specific and complex questions about how much hay he fed his horses and why. The next, he could barely tell me how old he was. I could see immediately that his behavior was not consistent with APD. But it was also inconsistent with mental retardation of the degree that he had been diagnosed with. Frankly, I really wasn't sure what I was dealing with, as I had never seen this particular pattern before.

To get a second opinion, I grabbed the school psychologist, whose office was adjacent to mine. She, too, conversed with Randy at some length, after which we excused ourselves and went into the hallway to talk. She said succinctly, "There's no way that kid has an IQ of sixty-eight. Beyond that, though, I don't know what you've got there."

More out of curiosity than because of any real suspicion of APD, I proceeded with central auditory testing. Sure enough, Randy's results were consistent with his documented cognitive ability: he had no pattern of deficit whatsoever but, rather, performed poorly on all of the measures I administered. Instead of stopping there, however, I decided to look more closely at Randy's patterns of performance *within* each test I had given him. This analysis revealed a very interesting finding. Randy would respond correctly to five or six items in a row, then miss the next five or six, then respond correctly again to the next five or six, and so on. This had occurred during every test I had administered. Next, I gave him a test that assessed his ability to sustain auditory attention over an extended time—the Auditory Continuous Performance Test (ACPT), developed by Dr. Robert Keith. In this test, the listener is told to pay attention to a monotonous (and long) presentation of words and to raise a thumb whenever the word *dog* is heard. People with attention-related deficits often show errors of omission (missing *dog* when it occurs) or impulsivity (raising a thumb when *dog* is not heard). Some people with AD/HD also show worsening performance over time, doing much better at the beginning of the test than near the end when the ability to sustain attention has been taxed to its fullest.

When his actual calculated number of errors of omission, impulsivity, or beginning-ending comparison was considered, Randy showed no pattern on this test either. But the overall score was poor, and when his behavior within the test was analyzed, I saw the same type of puzzling on-again, off-again performance that I had previously observed during central auditory testing. It appeared to be cyclical behavior that had a very clear pattern over time.

I had been right that Randy did not exhibit APD. His mother had also been right—mental retardation did not explain Randy's difficulties. When his pattern of performance—not just across tests, but *within* tests—was analyzed, Randy clearly showed rapid cycles of function and then dysfunction. These cycles could not be explained by auditory-based deficit, global cognitive deficit, or even attention deficit. Instead, I suspected a neurologic cause.

I referred Randy to a neurologist and friend in the area who quickly diagnosed Randy's difficulty—he was experiencing rapidly cycling, regular seizures in his brain. Randy's seizures, which occurred every couple of minutes or so (corresponding to his "off" times during testing), were very subtle. He simply missed what was going on around him for a few seconds. The frequency and regularity of Randy's seizures affected virtually all his testing to the same degree, explaining why Randy had tested the same each and every time. Because he had never experienced more disruptive and obvious seizures, this type of neurologic disorder had never been suspected. I also suspect that the lack of quality services—both medical and educational—in Randy's area, combined with other social and economic factors, assured that Randy would fall through the cracks. When appropriately medicated, however, Randy demonstrated that his cognitive capacity was, indeed, within the average range. As his mother had asserted all along, Randy was not mentally retarded.

I should emphasize that my own testing for central auditory dysfunction was not what led to Randy's finally being accurately diagnosed. He should never have seen me at all. His behavior and presenting difficulties were not consistent with APD, and my testing showed no pattern indicative of APD. Nothing in my tests shed light on Randy's situation. Rather, the way I interpreted Randy's behavior—behavior that would have been present during any type of testing, including the cognitive testing that he had undergone three times prior to my having seen him—assisted in understanding his disorder.

All too often, we professionals rely solely on what the scores on a test tell us. Test scores are important. Diagnosis and analysis of performance are dependent on the scores in a test. But we should always be aware that the child's or adult's behavior *during* the testing may provide information that is even more important than the final scores. We should always be on the lookout for patterns *within,* as well as *across,* tests that may help us understand *why* a person is having difficulties. In Randy's case, his rapidly cycling seizure activity was so regular and subtle that the clinician who had administered all three of his cognitive assessments had simply missed it. As a result, Randy had been deprived of an education—indeed, an entire life—because, at seventeen, there really was no hope that Randy would progress beyond vocational training before being dismissed from the educational system when he turned twenty-one.

Randy's case was extreme, and I have never seen quite such a blatant and dramatic example of misdiagnosis before or since. However, I have seen cases in which not all of the information has been integrated in a multidisciplinary fashion. In many of these cases, inappropriate diagnoses (APD among them) have been made while the true cause of the difficulty has gone undetected. I have also seen cases in which an appropriate diagnosis has been made, but with no attempt to determine how all the pieces of the puzzle fit together to describe the patterns of difficulty for a given person. As a result, management took a shotgun approach based on what types of difficulties *might* be experienced rather than being based either on any firm theoretical framework or on the unique needs of the person.

It is important to look for patterns that make sense both from a scientific and from a functional and behavioral perspective. Models of APD attempt to recognize the heterogeneous nature of APDs by describing them in terms of patterns of findings that frequently co-occur and can be used to guide management efforts.

DIFFERENT TYPES OF APD

No one theoretical model of APD is universally accepted; however, APD and its various manifestations can be viewed from several popular frameworks. The Buffalo model, developed by Dr. Jack Katz of Buffalo, New York, focuses on the relationship between patterns of performance on specific tests of auditory processing and learning difficulties in children. Dr. Frank Musiek of Dartmouth Medical School has proposed a method of dividing auditory processing deficits into subgroups on the basis of underlying brain-based etiologies.

My own model of APD, developed in collaboration with my good friend and colleague Dr. Jeanane Ferre of Oak Park, Illinois, is based both on the underlying neurophysiology *and* the relationship among different types of APD and language, learning, and communication difficulties. Familiarly referred to as the Bellis/Ferre model, our framework consists of three primary, and two secondary, subtypes of APD. Each of our subtypes has a distinct biologic site of dysfunction and clearly delineated auditory, cognitive, learning, and language associated symptoms. The three primary subtypes consist of patterns of difficulty associated with right-, left-, and interhemispheric dysfunction. The two secondary subtypes may be thought of as riding that fine, gray line between audition and receptive language, and audition and executive (or organizational) function. They are included in our auditory model because both of them result in specific patterns of deficit on our tests of central auditory function and because they lead to significant auditory complaints. The Bellis/Ferre model is, like all current models of APD, a theoretical view that is not universally accepted. However, it has been shown to be quite useful in understanding the relationship between auditory processing and functional difficulties and in guiding efforts for management that cross discipline boundaries and address the overall presenting complaints of the child or adult. That having been said, let us now consider the Bellis/Ferre subtypes of APD.

Primary Subtypes. It should be emphasized that the information presented here should not be used for diagnostic purposes and is not intended to provide a cookie-cutter approach to this complex topic. Just as not every item on a list of general indicators of APD is applicable to every person with APD, you should never assume that all of the symptoms associated with a given subtype will be present in a person. Instead, these subtypes delineate findings across domains that all rely on the same general brain region(s) and that can, often do, but don't *always* coexist. Adults may not exhibit any of the learning, cognitive, or language symptoms described in these subtypes because they have already acquired those skills and competencies prior to the onset of their auditory difficulties. This is especially true of those with adult-onset APD due to aging or other factors. Therefore, their complaints and symptoms may be confined to those that are related to listening.

Auditory Decoding Deficit. Auditory Decoding Deficit is the "purest" subtype of APD and is often the classic example provided when describing APD. Some scientists believe this to be the only "true" APD. However, because many other brain regions are involved in auditory processing and many other types of auditory processes, I would consider that to be an unrealistically narrow view of Auditory Processing Disorder.

Auditory Decoding Deficit occurs when the language-dominant (usually left) hemisphere of the brain does not function properly. Specifically, the presumed site of dysfunction in this subtype is the primary auditory cortex, where precise speech-sound encoding takes place. Therefore, the auditory symptoms of Auditory Decoding Deficit frequently resemble those of hearing loss. Other signs and symptoms of left-hemisphere dysfunction also may be present. The primary findings associated with Auditory Decoding Deficit are outlined below.

POSSIBLE *listening complaints:*

- Mishearing words and other auditory discrimination difficulties, such as hearing "Have you got a dime?" instead of "Have you got the time?"

- Misunderstanding the linguistic *content* of a communication due to inefficient auditory closure abilities (difficulty filling in the "missing pieces" of a message)

- Difficulty hearing speech in backgrounds of noise (note: this is a hallmark symptom of virtually all types of APD, as well as many other nonauditory disorders, because any problem with listening will be more apparent in noisy or distracting environments)

- Behaving as if a hearing loss is present even if hearing sensitivity is normal

- Difficulty understanding rapid speakers or speakers who do not enunciate clearly

- Frequently asking for repetitions, such as saying "Huh?" or "What?" and indicating that the information was not "heard" in the first place (e.g., "I didn't hear you" versus "I didn't understand what you meant")

POSSIBLE *language-related symptoms:*

- Poor left-hemisphere language function, particularly in syntax (the structure of speech) and possibly semantics (the meaning of speech)

- Poor vocabulary abilities

- Articulation errors that appear to have an acoustic, rather than developmental, basis

- Expressive language often better than receptive language

POSSIBLE learning- or academic-related symptoms:

- Reading and spelling difficulties in phonemic decoding (phonics and word-attack skills, or the sound portion of sound-symbol association)

- Poor sound blending, segmentation, and other phonological awareness abilities

- Poor invented-spelling abilities in lower grades

- Poor reading comprehension *resulting from* slow reading rate and poor word-attack skills

- Sight-word reading and spelling vocabulary significantly better developed

- Difficulty in classes that rely more on language and listening (e.g., social studies, language arts, lecture-based science classes, word problems in math) and better performance in nonauditory classes (e.g., mathematics calculation classes, including geometry, art, music)

- Better performance when verbally presented information is augmented with visual or multimodality cues

- Difficulty learning a foreign language (although a nonverbal, visual language, such as sign, may be learned more easily)

POSSIBLE cognitive findings:

- Better Performance (nonverbal) IQ than Verbal IQ

- Relative weaknesses in analytic (whole-to-part) skills and sequential processing

- Relative strengths in visual-spatial abilities, gestalt (part-to-whole) synthesis, object assembly, visual processing speed and accuracy, and related abilities

POSSIBLE associated symptoms:

- Typically, other modalities (visual, motor) are not involved

Results of central auditory testing show:

- Bilateral or right-ear deficit on dichotic tests (indicating left-hemisphere involvement) *combined with* poor perception of distorted or rapidly presented speech (auditory closure abilities)

- Poor fine-grained auditory discrimination (such as discriminating between *da* and *ga*)

- Electrophysiology *may be* abnormal in some cases, especially over the left hemisphere or when using measures involving speech-sound discrimination

Examples of Auditory Decoding Deficit discussed in this book:

- Jeff, Clay, Larry (chapter 1); Craig (chapter 3)

Prosodic Deficit. Prosodic Deficit may be thought of as the flip side of Auditory Decoding Deficit. That is, the left-hemisphere skills that represent areas of difficulty for the person with Auditory Decoding Deficit are usually areas of strength for the person with Prosodic Deficit. In addition, Prosodic Deficit, and other functional ramifications of right-hemisphere-based communication disorders, have only recently begun to be more commonly recognized and addressed in the literature. As a result, children and adults with Prosodic Deficit are frequently at risk of falling through the cracks because they may not exhibit significant enough difficulty to qualify for special education services under the classification of learning disability or language disorder and their symptoms may be far-reaching and more "emotionally" based. Furthermore, in many cases of Prosodic Deficit, the auditory complaints may be the least disruptive aspect of the overall disorder, and difficulties in other areas, including social judgment and emotional well-being, may require the greatest amount of attention. Because people with Prosodic Deficit often have these other, often more compelling, concerns in nonauditory areas, applying the label APD to them is possibly not really appropriate. Rather, it may be more appropriate to consider Prosodic Deficit as merely the auditory piece of a more global, right-hemisphere dysfunction. Thus, the APD portion of Prosodic Deficit is often a symptom, rather than the cause, of many of the person's functional difficulties.

The primary findings associated with Prosodic Deficit and, by definition, with right-hemisphere dysfunction, are outlined below.

POSSIBLE listening complaints:

- Misunderstanding the *intent* rather than the *content* of a communication, with the result that messages are frequently misinterpreted and hurt feelings often arise

- Difficulty understanding communication forms that rely on subtle changes in intonation, such as humor and sarcasm, as well as with words and sentences in which subtle differences in stress result in large differences in meaning (e.g., *con*vict versus con*vict*; *des*ert versus des*ert*; "*You* can't come with me!" versus "You can't come with *me!*")

- Difficulty extracting the key words from a message so that, even if a message can be repeated verbatim, the main idea is missed

- Good speech-sound discrimination and auditory closure abilities

- Feeling as if communications are heard perfectly well, but that they are not understood completely or, perhaps, that the speaker's tone of voice was inappropriate, rude, or insensitive

POSSIBLE *language-related symptoms:*

- Poor pragmatic abilities (i.e., poor *use* of language) and social communication skills, including inappropriate (or no) use of humor and frequent social faux pas

- Good syntax, semantics, articulation, and vocabulary skills

- Both expressive and receptive language abilities may technically be within the normal range on standardized testing

- Speaking quality may be monotonic or exhibit subtle differences in rate, stress, intonation, or fluency; facial affect may be "flat"

POSSIBLE *learning- or academic-related symptoms:*

- Poor sight-word reading and spelling abilities combined with intact phonics skills (difficulty with the symbol portion of sound-symbol association); using a phonological decoding strategy for words that should be within the sight-word vocabulary (trying to sound out words that should be familiar)

- Typically good phonological awareness abilities; however, sequencing may be an area of relative difficulty

- Good invented-spelling abilities in lower grades

- Poor reading comprehension resulting from slow reading rate due to inefficient sight-word abilities

- May have difficulty in classes that rely on language and listening due to difficulty with extracting the key words; however, greater difficulty is typically exhibited in classes such as mathematics (calculation, geometry), music, and art (difficulties with perspective may occur in drawing so that pictures unintentionally resemble Picassos)

- Learning a foreign language typically is not a problem; however, difficulty may arise when trying to learn visual languages (such as American Sign Language)

- Augmentation with visual or multimodality cues may have no effect on performance *or* they may assist if they graphically display the main intent of the message

POSSIBLE cognitive findings:

- Better Verbal IQ than Performance (nonverbal) IQ

- Relative weaknesses in gestalt (part-to-whole) synthesis and simultaneous processing, visual-spatial abilities, object assembly, visual processing speed and accuracy, and related abilities

- Poor abstract reasoning, but good understanding of concrete concepts

- Relative strengths in analytic (whole-to-part) skills and sequential processing; however, sequencing of responses may be an area of weakness

- Difficulties may be subtle enough that performance on standardized tests of learning and cognition may be relatively normal so that eligibility criteria for special education under a learning disabilities category are not met; alternatively, may meet criteria for a nonverbal learning disability

POSSIBLE associated symptoms:

- Psychological disturbances, including depression, may be a primary concern

- Attention-related deficits may be present due to inefficient right-hemisphere mechanisms for allocation of attention

- Some children with signs and symptoms of Prosodic Deficit may actually fall within the autistic spectrum; therefore, it is important not to attribute all difficulties such as those described here to primary APD

Results of central auditory testing show:

- Left-ear deficits on dichotic speech tasks (which can be indicative of either right- or interhemispheric dysfunction) *combined with* difficulty perceiving, humming, *and* labeling nonverbal tonal stimuli (i.e., difficulty hearing the subtle pitch or duration differences and the acoustic contour of the tonal pattern)

- Good fine-grained auditory discrimination (such as discriminating between *da* and *ga*)

- Electrophysiology *may be* abnormal in some cases, especially over the right hemisphere

Examples of Prosodic Deficit discussed in this book:

- The author (preface); Jason (chapter 1); Rose (chapter 4)

Integration Deficit. Our final primary subtype involves neither the left nor the right hemisphere of the brain. Instead, the way in which the two hemispheres interact and communicate with one another is affected. Because interhemispheric integration is required for so many different types of tasks and abilities spanning all modalities, the behavioral symptoms of Integration Deficit vary hugely from one person to another. For some, the auditory difficulties that accompany interhemispheric dysfunction may be the most disruptive. For others, difficulties in other modalities may be of more concern. Therefore, once again, it is important to recognize that the APD subtype that we refer to as Integration Deficit may represent merely one aspect of the person's overall difficulties, and that all of the person's complaints cannot and should not be attributed solely to an auditory deficit.

The primary findings associated with Integration Deficit are outlined below.

POSSIBLE *listening complaints:*

- Difficulty connecting the linguistic (or language-based) content with the prosodic (or tone-of-voice) intent of the message so that misunderstandings of the overall meaning of the communication occur (e.g., not responding correctly to "We're going to the movies tonight?" because the language implies a statement yet the tone of voice indicates that this is a question requiring a yes-or-no response)

- Significant difficulty hearing in noise because of the need for both ears (and both hemispheres of the brain) to work together to extract a signal from a noisy background

- Good speech-sound discrimination and specific auditory-closure skills

- Feeling either as if communications are not heard clearly or that they are not understood completely, depending on the situation

POSSIBLE *language-related symptoms:*

- Typically good syntax, semantics, vocabulary, and pragmatics when each is tested individually

- Both expressive and receptive language abilities are often within the normal range on standardized testing

POSSIBLE *learning- or academic-related symptoms:*

- Both sight-word and word-attack reading and spelling abilities may be affected because of a difficulty in the association portion of sound-symbol association, leading to slow reading rate, low reading accuracy, and ultimately, poor reading comprehension

- Typically good phonological awareness abilities

- May have difficulty in classes that rely on language and listening *and* in classes that are not auditory/verbal, depending on the particular task demands of each class

- Music abilities may be affected because of the need to link the "language" of musical notation with the melodic aspects; particular difficulty may be seen when trying to play instruments that require bimanual coordination (e.g., piano, in which each hand is doing something different based on different forms of notation—bass and treble clefs)

- Performance in PE may be poor due to difficulty with bimanual and bipedal coordination

- Augmentation with multimodality cues often results in confusion rather than clarification

- Note-taking may be particularly difficult because of the division of attention between auditory and visual modalities it requires

- Specific isolated skills, such as math calculation, are often intact; however, when the skill is combined with another requiring a different type of processing (e.g., math calculation using algebraic language), difficulties may arise

POSSIBLE cognitive findings:

- Verbal and Performance IQ will likely be equally developed; however, specific weaknesses will be found in those subtests that require both hemispheres of the brain to work together

- When taken in isolation, both analytic (whole-to-part) and gestalt (part-to-whole) abilities will likely be intact

- Difficulties in a skill area may be apparent during one type of task and not during another, simply because of the different demands of the tasks (rather than problems with the skill area); therefore, performance may seem inconsistent unless task demands are considered

POSSIBLE associated symptoms:

- Bimanual and bipedal coordination difficulties may occur, and sports may be difficult

- Possible attention-related concerns may be present due to difficulties with regulation of attentional resources between the hemispheres, a task that relies, at least in part, on the corpus callosum

- Visual-motor and visual-auditory integration deficits are often present

Results of central auditory testing show:

- Left-ear deficits on dichotic speech tasks (which can be indicative of either right- or interhemispheric dysfunction) *combined with* difficulty labeling nonverbal tonal stimuli; however, the ability to hum tonal patterns will be intact (ruling out right-hemisphere dysfunction)

- Good fine-grained auditory discrimination

- Electrophysiology typically is normal, except for very specialized (and relatively uncommon) measures in which hemispheric responses to specific speech stimuli are studied

Examples of Integration Deficit discussed in this book:

- Tim (preface); Evelyn (chapter 1); Bryce, Ralph (chapter 4)

Secondary Subtypes In addition to the three primary subtypes of APD, the Bellis/Ferre model also delineates two additional subtypes. These secondary subtypes recognize the relationship between audition and higher-order language or organizational function. Higher-order cognitive, language, or related disorders can result in poor listening abilities that cannot truly be considered auditory deficits; however, the line between audition and some of these higher-order functions is ethereal at best. That's why our two secondary subtypes consist of co-occurring signs and symptoms that also include specific patterns of test findings on our central auditory assessment tools. Because of these auditory-based diagnostic findings, we consider these subtypes to be, at least in part, auditory in nature.

Associative Deficit. The first, Associative Deficit, may also be thought of as an auditory-based receptive language disorder. People with Associative Deficit often have difficulty with a variety of receptive language abilities, particularly with semantics, or the meaning of speech. They seem to hear just fine, can often repeat what was said verbatim, but have difficulty understanding the meaning of the message. This difficulty is more apparent with complex sentences and higher-level linguistic forms, such as passive and compound sentences and those that include various forms of temporal (before, after, first, then), spatial (on, under, within), and related concepts. It is also much more apparent with spoken language, and reading comprehension is usually much better. Word-finding difficulties may be apparent in some cases.

Children with Associative Deficit may perform adequately in school until they reach approximately the third grade, when the linguistic demands increase markedly. Typically, these children perform far more poorly in auditory- or language-based classes than in those with less emphasis on understanding verbal information. On tests of central auditory function, people with Associative Deficit demonstrate clear signs of left-hemisphere dysfunction (e.g., bilateral or right-ear deficit on dichotic speech tasks). However, their auditory-closure and speech-sound-discrimination abilities are quite good, which suggests that the primary auditory cortex is working properly. Most measures of electrophysiology usually result in normal findings; however, some less common electrophysiologic measures that look specifically at semantic processing may be abnormal. Therefore, the apparent site of dysfunction for Associative Deficit is the auditory association cortex, where meaning and sound comes together. Inefficient communication between primary and associative cortical regions may also be to blame in some cases. Therefore, Associative Deficit may be thought of as a receptive language disorder falling within the group of disorders collectively known as the aphasias that has a strong auditory component. Both Harold and Tracy, in chapter 2, exhibited Associative Deficit; however, Harold's disorder was more appropriately termed receptive aphasia.

Output-Organization Deficit. The other secondary subtype of APD involves the efferent, or outgoing, auditory system and/or perhaps the frontal lobes that control executive function. Because this type of APD primarily manifests itself in difficulty organizing and following through on verbally presented information, we call it Output-

Organization Deficit. People with Output-Organization Deficit often exhibit signs and symptoms of an expressive language disorder. They may have difficulty formulating complex sentences and responding to direct, verbally presented questions or multistep directions. Other types of organization or planning skills may also be involved, including fine and gross motor-planning difficulties. Their difficulties are usually much more apparent when they are asked to act on information or instructions that were presented verbally. They usually do better when the same instructions are written. This subtype is included in our discussion of APD because the difficulties that appear are most apparent in response to verbally presented information and because specific findings on auditory testing occur.

Many people with Output-Organization Deficit demonstrate difficulty on any central auditory task that requires the report of more than two critical elements. Furthermore, contralateral acoustic reflexes (a measure of the auditory system's ability to respond to loud sounds by contracting tiny muscles in the middle ear) are often absent in Output-Organization Deficit, indicating that the auditory system is, indeed, involved to some degree. Similar to many other APDs, a hallmark symptom of Output-Organization Deficit is severe difficulty hearing in noise, a task for which the efferent auditory system, as well as many other regions of the central auditory pathways, is involved. Finally, Output-Organization Deficit frequently coexists with (or is merely an associated symptom of) higher-order executive function disorders, including AD/HD.

Other Forms of APD I should mention that other types of auditory processing disorders do exist that are not included in our primary or secondary subtypes. One of these that has received a great deal of recent interest is *auditory neuropathy,* a deficit in the ability of the fibers of the auditory nerve (or perhaps lower brain-stem neurons) to fire synchronously. People with auditory neuropathy exhibit clear physiologic findings, including abnormal auditory electrophysiology at the level of the auditory nerve or brain stem; very poor speech perception abilities, especially in noise; and possible hearing loss of virtually any degree, from mild to profoundly deaf. A specific diagnostic finding in auditory neuropathy is normal inner-ear function as measured by otoacoustic emissions. It is estimated that perhaps as much as 10 percent of congenital (present at birth) deafness or hearing loss may be due to auditory neuropathy.

"Central deafness" can be thought of as another type of auditory processing disorder. This rare condition results from damage to or dysfunction in the auditory cortex regions of both sides of the brain. People with central deafness, like those with auditory neuropathy, demonstrate normal inner-ear function on otoacoustic emission testing. Electrophysiologic measures of brain stem function are also normal. However, these same measures of function at higher brain (cortex) levels reveal abnormal or absent responses to sound. Behaviorally, people with cortical deafness truly are just that: deaf. But the deafness arises from dysfunction in the brain, not in the ear, auditory nerve, or brain stem.

With our model of APD, cognitive, learning, language, and related evaluations can be combined with results of central auditory testing to reveal specific patterns that suggest different subtypes of APD. Although the behavioral symptoms of each type of APD may be present to some degree in many other nonauditory disorders, each of these subtypes shows up clearly in patterns on diagnostic tests of central auditory function. Therefore, it is crucial that appropriate diagnostic measures of central auditory function be administered in any suspected case of APD. This is important, even if all behavioral symptoms seem to suggest the presence of APD, so that the presence of an actual auditory deficit can be confirmed and the type of deficit determined. Most important, management of the disorder will be based directly on the specific auditory deficit that is discovered.

WHEN A LISTENING PROBLEM IS *NOT* APD

By this point, you may be convinced that everyone you know has APD. After all, who among us has not had experience with someone who is a poor listener, does not follow directions well, or misunderstands what we mean or say? In the field of APD, as in many other professional arenas, too much knowledge can sometimes be a dangerous thing. I am concerned that, because of the common nature of many of the behavioral symptoms of APD, the disorder will become (or has already become) a generic, catchall diagnosis that will automatically be applied to anyone with listening problems, not unlike what has occurred with some active children and AD/HD.

Something else that concerns me greatly is the present popularity of the APD label. I have counseled many parents of children with significant language, cognitive, or related disorders who are hoping against hope for a diagnosis of APD. Some of them may even believe that APD is the true culprit underlying their children's difficulties, in spite of clear evidence to the contrary.

Someone may embrace and cling desperately to the diagnosis of APD without obtaining confirmation for many reasons. APD may seem relatively nonthreatening and innocuous compared to other disorders that can manifest themselves similarly. Some of these disorders are rather intimidating, especially those that have negative connotations. A disorder that "merely" affects how someone is hearing sounds is far more preferable, and far less threatening, than diagnoses such as mental retardation, AD/HD, or autism. I have seen many parents whose children have been accurately diagnosed with autism or mental retardation, yet who continue to search for more acceptable alternatives, such as APD.

Then there are cases in which no clear-cut answer has or even can be obtained. For some children with language, learning, or communication difficulties, we simply never really understand the reason why, so a diagnosis of APD is latched onto.

Laypersons and professionals may also adopt a diagnosis of APD without confirmation because of the lack of comprehensive and accurate information about APD. Although books and articles on APD have been published, most of them have been written for the scientist or communication-disorders professional. Many of them are difficult to understand even for clinicians in my own field. Few resources exist for the person outside of the arena of speech and hearing. As a result, there is a general lack of awareness of how APD can manifest itself in various, methods of diagnosing APD, and methods of treating it. Instead, many laypersons and professionals must rely on incomplete, grossly generalized, and sometimes even outright inaccurate information. Information such as that presented in chapters 2 and 3 of this book may be available in condensed, checklist style to the general reader; however, the true complexity of the disorder cannot possibly be dealt with in this type of abbreviated manner. But that is all many concerned parents, professionals, and others have had available to them—which was a key motivation for me to write the book that you now hold in your hands.

Finally, and perhaps most importantly, the reported instances of "miracle cures" or therapy techniques that alleviate a child's difficulties seemingly overnight provide an irresistible temptation for parents and others looking for answers. Many clinics—including my own—are filled with parents demanding a specific therapy technique or program because they have heard that it worked for other children with similar difficulties to their own child's. In no area of medicine, learning, communication disorders, or any other field is there one therapy or treatment that will "cure" everyone, regardless of the nature of the underlying disorder. No matter how attractive it seems, such an idea is simply not plausible. Yet, much of the information available in the public domain on the subject of APD seems to promise just such simple answers.

Auditory Problems as Symptoms I've said it before and I'll say it again: not all listening difficulties can be attributed to APD, no matter how similar some of the symptoms seem. People with attention deficits, language or cognitive disorders, or other types of dysfunction will likely be poor auditory processors (or listeners), but not because of an actual disorder in the auditory system per se. Rather, something else is impacting their auditory abilities on a higher level in a top-down fashion so that the auditory difficulties are a symptom rather than the cause of the person's difficulties.

These groups of people usually have two primary things in common: (1) they have listening problems of some type that can't be attributed to any actual auditory deficit, and (2) they typically demonstrate no clear pattern of performance (or completely normal scores) on diagnostic tests of central auditory processing. Let's take a look at just some of these conditions that may look like APD but are not.

Disorders affecting procedural memory. Some people have difficulty following daily routines. Whether we consider the absentminded professor who cannot remember to tie his shoes in the morning, the elderly gentleman suffering from early dementia, or the child with global memory problems, deficits in such procedural memory, or memory for routine procedures, are not a hallmark of APD. When I see people who exhibit some of the classic symptoms of APD, such as difficulty following directions and understanding information presented in the classroom, I always check to see how they do with daily routines. If, for example, the child cannot remember where to put his coat in the morning (despite having been told to place it in the same spot since the beginning of school and it is now spring!), I begin to suspect some higher order cognitive or memory deficit rather than an auditory-based disorder. People with APD typically have difficulty with novel information, but do well with information or routines that are already learned.

Neurologic and psychological disorders. When a person is focusing internally on something other than the conversation at hand, we would not expect him or her to comprehend and retain all of what is being said. We have all had our minds wander during a conversation, only to have something (such as a direct question requiring a response) snap us back to the present. Then we realize that we have absolutely no idea what our conversational partner is talking about. Usually, we are forced to admit that we were "somewhere else," and we ask the person to repeat what was said. Episodes like this occur for all of us, but they are much more frequent in some disorders. For example, certain psychological disorders, by definition, disconnect the person from reality. Seizure disorders can cause information to be missed during a seizure and may be very subtle behaviorally. Children with autism may exhibit poor auditory skills, but they also exhibit other, nonauditory symptoms such as stereotyped and repetitive routines or "scripts" that they adhere to; motor mannerisms (often referred to as self-stimulating behaviors) such as hand-flapping, rocking, or finger-snapping; poor use of nonverbal social communication behaviors such as eye contact; and similar behaviors. Thus, when these types of behaviors are seen in a child, it is unreasonable to assume that an underlying auditory deficit is to blame. People with bipolar disorders may also exhibit sensory, including auditory, processing difficulties because of difficulty transitioning between and regulating states of attention in response to incoming environmental stimuli. Many conditions may result in APD-like symptoms, but the presence of other, nonauditory behaviors is an important clue that APD is not primary.

Attention disorders. The one disorder that may most closely resemble and be confused with APD is attention-deficit/hyperactivity disorder. AD/HD can occur in three forms: with hyperactivity, without hyperactivity (or predominantly inattentive), or mixed. Any of these forms of AD/HD will affect a person's ability to listen. As a result, persons with AD/HD and APD can demonstrate many of the same listening behaviors, including distractibility, difficulty following verbal directions, and similar complaints. Moreover, APD and AD/HD fre-

quently coexist, with the result that the attention deficit makes the auditory deficit much more disruptive. We must attempt to separate the
effects of each of these disorders, and to obtain appropriate treatment
for the attention deficit before addressing the auditory disorder. This
is the only way our auditory management can be most efficient and
effective.

Language disorders. Any condition that affects receptive language
ability will affect listening comprehension skills. APD is only one of
these conditions. Children and adults may exhibit primary language
disorders due to unknown causes or that are the result of stroke or
head trauma. These disorders should not be included under the "APD
umbrella." Although it is difficult at times to separate language processing from auditory processing, some clues can help us do so. For example, the child who exhibits good word-attack skills, sight-word
skills, reading rate and accuracy, auditory discrimination, and all of
those other auditory-based bottom-up abilities, but who, nevertheless,
has difficulty comprehending the information, may well have a
language, rather than an auditory, deficit. Similarly, people who are
communicating in a nonnative language will understandably have
comprehension difficulties that cannot properly be termed a disorder.
When language, rather than audition, is to blame, our therapy time
will be much more well spent if we focus on the language-related issues rather than on bottom-up, auditory-based input skills.

General memory disorders. Many of the children I see for central auditory evaluation or consultation do not exhibit listening difficulties
per se. Instead, they have problems following through with what is expected of them. For these children, and adults like them, the primary
cause of their difficulties is not APD. Instead, these people *hear* what is
said, *understand* the meaning, but then, for whatever reason, fail to initi-
ate and/or complete the task. We have all had the experience of walking to another room only to forget what it was we were going for once

we arrive. When this type of behavior is pervasive or frequent, the possibility of a higher order memory, cognitive, or attention disorder should be explored, rather than placing the blame on an auditory-based deficit.

Behavior disorders. Let's face it, sometimes even the most compliant of people will demonstrate what is commonly referred to as selective listening. These people hear only what they want to hear and ignore the rest. Some children are experts at selective listening. They never seem able to hear when they are asked to set the table. They can't carry on even the simplest of conversations if a favorite cartoon is on television. Yet, they can both detect and understand any conversation, no matter how quietly conducted, regarding a proposed trip to their favorite fast-food restaurant at one hundred paces even in a background of noise. Their auditory processing skills are entirely intact. These types of behaviors are common in everyone, although some exhibit them more often than others. In addition, psychological disorders such as oppositional defiant disorder and conduct disorder can also result in lack of follow-through on instructions or directions that may resemble APD. It is important to separate behavioral or psychological factors from those that are specifically auditory-related and to address the nonauditory factors.

Hearing loss. No discussion of APD in children or adults would be complete without mentioning hearing loss once again. Ruling out even the most mild or transient of hearing losses should be the absolute first step any time APD is suspected, whether in a child or an adult. Minimal or fluctuating hearing loss in a child with chronic ear infections will certainly affect that child's auditory skills and may lead to more persistent language, auditory, and learning difficulties later on if not addressed. Hearing loss in adults will also resemble APD. APD and hearing loss can coexist, and a hearing loss will exacerbate any auditory processing difficulty. Management of the hearing loss should be undertaken prior to focusing on the more central auditory processing factors.

It is not enough merely to suspect the presence of an auditory processing deficit. No matter how much a person's difficulties resemble those of APD, it may not be APD at all. Appropriate diagnosis is critical both to achieve an understanding of the nature of the disorder and to determine how the disorder fits in with the other learning, cognitive, communication, and related difficulties a given person is experiencing. Only then can APD be treated appropriately.

6

TREATING APD

NO MATTER HOW much knowledge you have about APD, no matter how many quality services are available in your area, and no matter what specific type of APD is present and how it affects daily functioning, none of this information is worth a thing unless you can do something about the disorder. Unfortunately, no one treatment, management approach, or intervention will cure all cases of APD, no matter how badly we wish this to be the case. Auditory processing deficits are complex. APD and the way in which it affects daily life are different from one person to the next. So, too, must the management approach developed be individualized for each person with APD.

We know that the brain is plastic, that it can be changed with stimulation (or lack thereof) so that deficient skill areas may be rehabilitated. But the degree to which treatment will be effective cannot be predicted for any given person. Some people with APD, especially young children, eventually catch up after rehabilitation and no longer manifest signs, symptoms, or diagnostic indicators of the disorder. Others, however, have less success with remediation techniques and may continue to have problems in certain listening, learning, or communicative situations throughout their lives. This is why management of APD focuses not just on remediating the disorder, but also on managing the listening environment and on teaching methods of compensating.

THE GRIEVING PROCESS

One important topic that has direct bearing on our ability to manage and remediate APD is the grief that often accompanies the diagnosis of a disability, any disability. Even when a diagnosis of APD is accompanied by a sense of relief—relief at finally knowing what the problem is, relief that it is not something infinitely worse—grief is an unavoidable by-product. And it can take many forms. For the adult who is newly diagnosed with APD, anger and denial may predominate, leading to assertions that there is no problem at all. Some adults with APD may insist that the fault for communication difficulties lies with others or that rehabilitation would be a waste of time. Much of the immediate postdiagnosis counseling with adults includes educating them about the disorder, the rationale underlying rehabilitative efforts, and the need to involve family and significant others in the management process. First and foremost, however, counseling must focus on helping the person accept the presence of the disorder.

Parents of children diagnosed with disabilities, including APD, may experience serious and pervasive grief that can last a long time. The stages of this grief are not unlike those delineated by Elisabeth Kübler-Ross in her book *On Death and Dying*. First, there is anger—anger at the professionals, especially if misdiagnoses have occurred, anger at themselves and each other, even anger at God for allowing such an event. Even if the professionals have arrived at an accurate diagnosis early in the process, and no misconduct is apparent, parents tend, nevertheless, to blame them for perceived missteps. The natural instinct is for parents to focus their overwhelming emotions toward the bearers of the bad news because the need to strike out at someone or something is all-encompassing.

Next, there is denial. It doesn't matter if parents have suspected some type of disorder; denial is a normal and inevitable step in the grieving process. This is to be expected. The confirmation of a disorder or disability means that their child is not like all of the other "normal" children. This realization can be devastating. So the first reaction may be to pretend that nothing at all is wrong. This is especially true when the disorder or disability can't be seen, as is the case with hearing loss or APD.

Sometimes denial takes the form of lack of follow-through on recommendations. This inactivity may be rationalized by such statements as "My child is just fine, the professionals are wrong" (even when the parent was the one who suspected the disorder in the first place) or "I had similar problems when I was a kid, too, but I caught up. So will my child." Denial can also manifest itself in seeming disinterest. The parents may not appear to listen to advice or read information provided. It is as if their emotional systems are on overload and they cannot possibly take any more in without exploding. At other times, denial takes the opposite form: becoming obsessed with gathering as much information as possible as quickly as possible. Parents may desire to shop around for a new diagnosis, a second or third or fourth opinion, or a promise of treatment that will cure the disorder overnight and take away the need to deal with the brutal reality.

I frequently see this latter form of denial in my own practice, and it often leads to the "bandwagon phenomenon" whenever a new therapy approach appears in the scientific or popular literature. When any new approach has been shown to be successful with some children, parents may jump on the bandwagon to demand the exact same therapy for their own child, convinced that it will work for him or her, too. They may not understand that no therapeutic technique is appropriate for all children. They may not see the differences (in characteristics, type of deficit, or diagnosis) between their own child and the ones who have benefited from the new therapy. Often, they refuse to hear explanations about the need for appropriate diagnosis, descriptions of other therapy approaches that may be far more appropriate for their child, or caveats that their child's disorder is not likely to be completely remediated by the therapy. Instead, the new therapy approach represents an opportunity to take away the disorder entirely, as if it never existed at all. This type of denial often fosters unrealistic expectations.

I have also seen the same type of bandwagon phenomenon occur with the diagnosis of APD itself. Sometimes parents will hear or read of a child who had been diagnosed with autism (or mental retardation or another disorder) and who was ultimately found to have APD instead. The parents may then become convinced that their own child (also diagnosed with autism or mental retardation) has APD, even if a diagnosis of APD is neither likely nor appropriate. In my experience, this has been a leading reason for the dramatic upsurge we've seen recently in inappropriate requests or referrals for APD evaluation and treatment services. For some parents, APD may represent an opportunity to deny their child's real disorder in favor of one less threatening.

Denial may also cause parents to hear only what they want to hear and to unconsciously discard information that is discouraging. Thus, a parent may focus on one sentence, gesture, or expression and ignore the context in which it occurred. For example, if the clinician says, "This therapy approach is often effective for the type of disorder your child has," the parent may hear, "This therapy approach will cure your child." Conversely, if other associated disorders are even mentioned, such as AD/HD or autism, as in "I have found this behavioral technique to be useful for children with APD, as well as those with autism or AD/HD," parents may react defensively, absolutely convinced that the obvious implication in the statement was that *their* child was autistic or had AD/HD, even if the clinician intended no such thing. This absolute conviction and distortion of reality may have an adverse impact on the ability of the parents and the clinician to work together effectively as a team and may persist for years after a conversation.

It is important to realize that this, as with all stages of grief, is normal and to be expected. Indeed, this form of denial is necessary because there is only so much that we, as humans, can cope with at any time. So much information is being provided during diagnosis and counseling that it is sometimes impossible for a parent not to narrow the focus, to attend to a select number of issues at a time. Also, parents may just not be ready to hear some things, particularly that associated disorders are possible or that some difficulties may remain even after therapy is concluded. As a professional, I have learned to expect this, and I know that much of the information I provide will need to be repeated over time before it can be understood and assimilated.

All too often, diagnosis of a disorder is made without providing parents with ample time to digest the input and devise questions. Frequently, all of the critical information is provided at once. What parents may not, at first, be ready to hear—the degree to which their child is delayed in speech or language, the potential learning ramifications—may be entirely acceptable when broached later or by another professional. The importance of individualized counseling over several sessions cannot be overemphasized.

Bargaining and depression may also occur. Bargaining, which may consist of everything from pleas to higher powers ("I'll never argue with my husband again, I swear, God, if you'll just make this better") to more earthbound goals ("I'll learn everything I can about this disorder and I'll do anything, pay anything, travel anywhere, to fight this thing"), may often be beneficial in some ways. That is, it is often at this point that parents become truly involved in the management of their child's disorder, following through on suggestions learned during therapy. On the other hand, parents sometimes become so involved in their child's disorder that everything and everyone else is excluded, even other family members. The disorder becomes the sole focus of their lives. In addition, the sometimes helpful—but often incomplete—information that parents may obtain from a variety of sources sometimes results in what I call "therapy bombardment." So many different therapy approaches are pursued simultaneously—some appropriate and reasonable, some not—that the child is pulled in many different directions at once. As a result, the effectiveness of each approach is minimized. As a parent, I understand the need to protect and advocate for my child and to explore every avenue available. But my clinical experience has taught me that, when this is carried to excess, the result may be more harmful than helpful. In some cases it may be detrimental to family relationships, interactions with the clinician, and even the emotional well-being of the parents and the child. Yet again, it is important to recognize that this is a normal, understandable stage of grieving that many parents must go through before they can move on.

Warring with such bargaining tendencies, and sometimes alternating with them in a dizzying roller coaster of emotions, is depression. Many parents I work with report that, on one day (or at one moment), they feel ready to sally forth and take on the entire world on behalf of their child. The next moment, however, they want nothing more than to crawl under a blanket in a dark room, let loose the tears, and drift into oblivious sleep. The what-ifs roll relentlessly through their mind: What if I hadn't drunk coffee or the occasional alcoholic drink during my pregnancy? What if I hadn't worked up until my due date? What if we had insisted that the doctor refer us for an evaluation sooner? What if I had read all those baby books and recognized that my baby wasn't developing normally? What if my husband (or wife) hadn't convinced me that nothing was wrong? What if? What if? What if? And, the most difficult what-if of all—one that crosses many parents' minds inadvertently at least once and for which they may feel guilt almost beyond bearing: What if my child had never been born?

Again, these are normal, entirely understandable responses to the diagnosis of a disability in a child. Nothing can make them go away completely, nothing can be done to avoid them entirely. And many of them are unavoidable consequences of parenthood, in general. Every parent, even those whose children exhibit no disorder or disability, ask themselves what-if questions. All of us worry about what our child will grow up to be and do, how well adjusted he or she will be, how successful, how happy. But when a child has a disability, these concerns are intensified.

When depression becomes pervasive and symptoms such as constant lethargy or sleeping too much, eating too much, self-imposed isolation, and inability to rouse oneself and carry on daily tasks occur, psychological counseling should be obtained. Parents must take steps to help themselves so that they, in turn, can help their child.

It can be a long road, but the final stage of the grieving process can be reached: acceptance. Acceptance is not giving in to the disorder. It is an open acknowledgment of the nature and ramifications of the disorder, and the need for appropriate intervention. Acceptance means adopting realistic expectations of what the outcome of any therapy program may be, while retaining hope for the best possible result. Acceptance means shifting focus away from the child's disorder alone and back to the child in his or her entirety and to the family as a unit.

Be aware, however, that although I have laid out each step in an orderly sequence, grief doesn't really work that way. Some parents may skip entire stages in grieving, go through them in a different order, or experience more than one at once. Others may find themselves stuck at one point—for example, denial or bargaining—and never reach acceptance. Still others may find themselves finally and blessedly able to accept, only to revisit earlier stages each time the child reaches a new point in development or education and new problems arise: the beginning of elementary school, middle school, high school, college. The announcement of each new therapeutic technique may trigger the entire process all over again. And anger may rise up without warning at any time.

I have worked with many parents of high-school-aged children with APD who, for the first time, are experiencing and expressing anger. Often their anger is directed toward those professionals who worked with the child and "missed" the diagnosis (despite that little was known about APD several years ago). These parents are angry over the years lost and the therapy that belatedly proved effective (but was unavailable when their children were much younger). Parental depression and guilt may persist, albeit subtly, even when the child reaches adulthood, with the person with the disorder given special treatment over other siblings, which can disrupt family dynamics. Thus, the process of grieving is many layered and may never completely be ended.

Even more devastating to the family is that both parents rarely experience the same stage of grieving at the same time. In the vast majority of families with whom I consult, one parent is far more receptive to hearing what I have to say than is the other. The most common scenario I encounter is that one parent (often the mother but not always) becomes an active participant in the management program of the child while the other parent continues to deny that anything is wrong. In extreme cases, this disparity can lead to separation, even divorce.

I am often asked to intervene in these situations, to convince the obstinate partner to see the light. But this is something I cannot do. Each person must go through the grieving process in his or her own time, in his or her own way. There are no absolutes. There are no rules. There is no right and wrong. Grieving just *is*, and it is different for every person. Parents need to allow themselves the time, the support (professional, if needed), and the freedom to feel. And professionals such as myself need to respect those needs and to accommodate them in every way possible as we work together to help the child.

Parents are uniquely attuned to the state of their child. Even without courses in child development, they know instinctively when something is wrong. As a professional, I have learned to trust their instincts. Although many parents, including myself, seem to constantly ask "Are you *sure* he's okay?" I have found that when a parent tells me that something is wrong with their child's hearing or speech development, the parent is usually right. Not only do parents sometimes recognize a disorder or disability long before anyone outside the family, a parent will frequently have a better handle on the nature of the problem—better even than the doctor.

But even when a parent is absolutely sure of the diagnosis before it is formally obtained, grief still occurs. Before they actually obtain an accurate diagnosis, all of the parents' attention and energies are focused on solving the mystery of what is wrong with their child. Once an accurate diagnosis has been obtained, however, grieving invariably begins.

Acknowledgment of the stages of grieving and how they may manifest themselves in parents of children with APD or in individuals with APD may be thought of as the first, and quite possibly most important, step in the management process. But several other components of APD management must be integral parts of any treatment program.

BASIC PRINCIPLES OF APD MANAGEMENT

Management of APD should incorporate three primary principles: (1) environmental modifications, (2) remediation (direct therapy) techniques, and (3) compensatory strategies. All three of these components are necessary for APD intervention to be effective. In addition, the details of each component should be deficit-specific; that is, they should be developed specifically for the person with APD and the unique circumstances of his or her learning or communicative difficulties and needs.

Environmental modifications consist of changing the learning or working environment so that access to verbally presented information is maximized. Remember, a child is in the classroom to learn, be it science, social studies, mathematics, or language arts. An adult is in the workplace to work, to get a job done, to further a career. These environments have their own intrinsic challenges. We do not want an additional challenge—such as coping with an auditory deficit—to interfere with the primary objectives of school or work. We don't want the person to be honing auditory skills when he or she should be focusing on learning the digestive system or developing an advertising campaign. Therefore, we must develop ways of making the information more accessible to the person with APD.

Remediation, on the other hand, should be challenging and should focus on the auditory deficit itself. Through clearly defined therapy techniques, we hope to train specific auditory and listening skills and change the way the brain processes auditory information, hopefully to ameliorate the disorder. The therapy environment should therefore be separate from the learning or work environment.

Finally, because some people with APD will continue to experience symptoms of their disorder even after remediation, it is important that they learn methods of living with the disorder. Thus, the teaching of compensatory strategies is an important, but often overlooked, component of the overall management program.

ALL THE WORLD'S A STAGE: ENVIRONMENTAL MODIFICATIONS AT SCHOOL

The first component of any APD management program should be to modify the environment. The modifications indicated will depend on whether the person with APD is in school, working for a living, or at home with family and friends. Remember, these environmental modifications are not intended to remediate, or fix, the disorder. They are employed to provide an environment that is user- (or listener-) friendly so that access to information is improved.

The classroom modifications that are appropriate will depend on the specific type of APD. Although preprinted lists of "classroom suggestions for children with APD" do exist, we should recognize that not all of the suggestions included on such lists are appropriate for *every* child with APD. In fact, some that are quite beneficial for most children with APD may actually be harmful or, at the very least, ineffective for others. Common school-based management strategies for children with APD follow.

Methods of Improving the Acoustic (or Listening) Environment

- **Pay special attention to seating.** Children with APD should be seated where they can see the teacher clearly and are away from distractions or noise. Any child can benefit from this advice. We all hear and understand better if we can see the speaker's face. Being able to see the speaker is critical for the child with virtually any type of APD. Don't assume, however, that the best seat in the class is always in the front row. If, for example, the front row is too close to the teacher, the child may find himself looking up at the teacher's chin rather than her face. And if the child is placed far away from the center of the front row so that only the side of the teacher's face is visible, the child will still have difficulties. The child with APD should sit as far back as he feels comfortable and off to the side up to about forty-five degrees, as long as the whole of the teacher's face is well lit and visible.

  For classes in which traditional rows of seats are not used (such as early-elementary-school classrooms in which desks may be in "pods" or small groups), finding the best seat can be more of a challenge. For instance, the teacher might designate a "speaker's throne" on which anyone (including the teacher) must sit when addressing the class. The throne can consist merely of a tall stool, and the children can decorate it in any way they like. The key is to place the throne in a spot where the child (or children) with APD can see the speaker clearly. This is a fun way of deciding preferential seating while not drawing undue attention to the child with APD. Some teachers have even reported that it brings more order to the class as a whole and increases turn-taking behavior and class participation. And it can give the tired teacher a chance to rest her legs during the day! Remember, however, that this trick may not work in all elementary classrooms. Preferential seating and how to implement it should be determined class by class.

Teachers who like to roam while talking may need to remain within a predetermined area. Children with APD should be seated so that they can see the teacher easily no matter where she goes within this space. Although some teachers may feel restricted at first, they soon become accustomed to giving important information and directions from their "stages." Once the information is given, they can roam about the room, offering individual words of encouragement or further direction to their students as needed.

At all times, teachers should pay attention to the lighting in the room. They should make sure that they are not standing in front of open windows and talking when they are backlit and their faces are in shadow. They should also make sure they are always facing the students when giving important information, rather than writing on the chalkboard or looking down at their notes.

Finally, special attention should be given to sources of noise in the room. The hum of a radiator, the whir of an overhead-projector fan, or the buzz of a fluorescent light may interfere with a child's ability to hear the teacher. Even if the child is seated where he can see the teacher well, the noise from these devices may negate any advantage from preferential seating. Either the device or the student should be moved.

- **Consider using an auditory trainer or other assistive listening device in the classroom.** The research is clear: all children in all classrooms benefit when they can hear the speaker clearly. Studies have shown that even children without learning or auditory deficits do better in classrooms that use amplification systems. In a perfect world, every classroom would have a sound-field amplification system installed. Children would be able to hear clearly without straining, and teachers' voices would be preserved. But this is not a perfect world, and the vast majority of children in our schools must contend with less-than-ideal listening conditions.

One of the most valuable aids for some children with APD is a personal amplification system to reduce background noise and allow the child to hear the teacher better. There are many different styles and types of these devices, referred to collectively as *assistive listening devices*. Although commonly recommended for children with APD, these devices may not be appropriate in many, even most, situations.

Schools should determine which children will benefit most from assistive listening technology. Schools have limited funds, and they must distribute those funds wisely so that every child can obtain the services he or she truly needs. Fitting every child who has APD with an assistive listening device may not only be ineffective in many cases, but may divert money from other areas in which it is needed more.

How, then, do we determine which children really need assistive listening technology to function in school? We must consider the nature of the auditory deficit in each child. For example, the child with Auditory Decoding Deficit is similar to the child with a hearing loss in that many portions of the message are missing or heard incompletely or inaccurately. For these children, the clarity of the acoustic signal is of paramount importance, and an assistive listening device is often appropriate.

On the other hand, the child with Prosodic Deficit has a type of auditory difficulty that is not related to the clarity of the signal. Even under ideal listening conditions, these children still have problems understanding intent and extracting the key words from a message. Use of assistive listening technology will usually not benefit the child with Prosodic Deficit any more than it benefits any other child in the classroom. Similarly, for the child with Associative Deficit, the primary issue is *meaning* rather than clarity. Again, even if the information is heard quite clearly, the child may be unable to understand it.

Children with Integration or Output-Organization Deficit

may experience significant difficulty hearing in noise. Assistive listening devices may help some of these children hear the information more clearly and may assist in learning. But, again, this decision should be made on an individual needs basis.

It is not enough merely to provide a child with an assistive listening device and assume that it will help the child listen and learn. Any child fitted with such a device should be monitored carefully to see if it is of benefit. Moreover, although hearing loss is unlikely, the child's hearing sensitivity should be tested regularly to make sure that no hearing loss is incurred from the use of the device. Finally, the device itself should be monitored to make sure that it remains in good working order. An assistive listening device that delivers a distorted signal or has a dead battery is no better—and probably worse—than no device at all.

When determining who should use assistive listening devices, we should also consider the age of the child. For the most part, assistive listening devices are accepted readily by children in elementary school. But once a child reaches middle or high school, priorities shift, and image becomes more important. Clothing, hairstyles, and jewelry take precedence over being able to hear clearly, especially if hearing clearly requires wearing something over the ears. Forcing the issue often leads to nothing but rebellion and a decrease in the adolescent's self-image. For these reasons, the use of personal assistive listening technology may be less appropriate and successful once a child reaches the later academic years.

Finally, I should mention that some other ear-related interventions, recommended by some professionals, may seem to make sense at first, but may actually be harmful. At one point, a frequent recommendation for children with APD was to plug one ear (usually the "weaker" or left ear) and allow the child to listen only through the right ear. This was usually recommended for children who exhibited left-ear deficits during dichotic listening tests. The inaccurate assumption was that, because the left ear was weaker during dichotic listening, only the right ear should be used during real-world listening. This assumption clearly reflects an incomplete or inaccurate understanding of the neurophysiology underlying binaural—or two-eared—listening. The use of an earplug in this manner is not recommended for children with APD. Indeed, this practice will likely be harmful to the child. Plugging one ear results in an undesirable reorganization of the auditory pathways. This practice, if followed consistently, may result in a worsening of binaural listening deficits that will persist long after the use of the earplug is discontinued.

Another potentially harmful practice I often see is children's use of assistive listening devices consistently in all classes and activities over many years. Although this may improve a child's access to information in the short term, it may have undesirable long-term results. The child may become overly dependent on the device and may lose (or simply never learn) the skills necessary for listening in real-world situations outside the school setting. Use of an assistive listening device should be carefully considered, and only for those classes or activities in which it is necessary. Children should have the opportunity to practice real-world listening during recess, physical education, music, and art classes. We must carefully balance the need to improve the acoustic clarity of the signal with the potential for overdependence on assistive listening devices. If children with APD are only given opportunities to listen and learn under ideal, amplified, artificial conditions, they may find themselves unable to listen or learn in the less-than-ideal real world.

- **Analyze the listening environment.** Certain classroom characteristics will make the room more listener-friendly to all students. These include carpeting on the floors, acoustic tiles on the ceilings, and the minimization of hard wall surfaces as much as possible. These characteristics help to reduce the amount of sound bouncing off floors, walls, and ceilings and decrease echoes (or *reverberation*) so that the signal is much clearer.

Schools with an open-classroom design—one in which partial walls are erected and noise spills over from adjacent classrooms—may be particularly inappropriate for children with APD. Because noise affects hearing even for children who do not have APD, many schools in this country have moved away from the open-classroom design, which was so popular a couple of decades ago. But this design remains, especially in some private or experimental schools or in school districts with limited funding.

The acoustic characteristics of every classroom should be analyzed carefully to ensure that children can hear the teacher clearly. If funding for changes is an issue, low-cost interventions such as the placement of cardboard egg cartons (empty, of course) on the ceilings and walls and inexpensive throw rugs on the floors can go a long way toward absorbing sound and reducing reverberation. Carpet squares, often available at little or no cost from the local carpet store's trash pile, offer a colorful, sound-absorbing alternative to hard walls. They can even be hung above partial walls in open classroom areas to decrease spillover of sound from adjacent rooms. Elementary-school students may enjoy decorating egg cartons or creating colorful banners to line the walls of the room. Making the room acoustically friendly can become a class art project that involves everyone, and the results can be as pleasing to the eye as to the ear.

Methods of Improving Students' Comprehension and Retention of Information

- **Make frequent checks for understanding.** Because children with APD often do not understand directions or instructions in the classroom, they should be monitored carefully to make sure that learning and comprehension are taking place. This does not mean asking "Do you understand?" in front of the entire class. Many children will nod their heads yes if asked this question point-blank, regardless of whether they understand the information. A better way of checking might be to ask the child to rephrase what has been said. Rephrasing, rather than merely repeating, is important because some children with APD can repeat verbatim an entire message, yet still not get it. This strategy is most appropriate and effective in one-on-one interactions with the child because, if used too frequently in front of the entire class, it draws attention to the child and perhaps sets her up for embarrassment.

An even better way of checking for understanding is to observe the child and see if she is doing what was required. If not, she can be redirected, gently and discreetly. Perhaps a secret sign can be developed between the teacher and the child—for example, moving a finger in a circle, meaning, "Look around you and see what the other children are doing"—to alert the child that she is not on task without disrupting the rest of the class. In this manner, the child also begins to learn an important compensatory strategy, that of carefully observing what is going on around her as a guide to her own performance and behavior.

- **Provide a note-taker.** Taking notes effectively is an important skill, usually taught in late elementary school or early middle school. Using a system of "guided note-taking," teachers can help students learn to identify key information in a lecture and organize it in written notes. Under these circumstances, it usually is the note-taking itself, not the information presented in the lecture, that is the important skill being learned. When note-taking is the focus of the lesson in school, children with APD will benefit from such instruction just as their classmates will. However, in later grades in which note-taking is not the focus of the lecture, but rather a tool designed to help the child remember information, note-taking can actually get in the way of learning the key information for some children with APD.

Note-taking requires a division of attention between auditory and visual modalities. When attention is focused on writing down information, less is available for listening to and comprehending the information in the first place. As a result of this division of attention, the child may neither hear the information nor write good, legible notes. In addition, for children with certain types of APD, note-taking relies on those very skills with which the child has great difficulty. For example, the child with inter-hemispheric Integration Deficit has difficulty with many cross-modality skills. Note-taking relies on listening and writing simultaneously, a task requiring both sides of the brain to work together effectively. The child with right-hemisphere Prosodic Deficit, on the other hand, may be unable to extract key words from the message, which is the essence of note-taking. Although the child with left-hemisphere Auditory Decoding Deficit may be able to take notes quite well, many of the words may be misspelled or the wrong words may be substituted because of the child's difficulty in hearing information clearly. These children are also trying to compensate for their auditory deficits by using their visual systems and watching the teacher's face. Note-taking requires them to look down at the page and to listen only with their ears, taking away the visual cues they rely on so heavily.

Children with Output-Organization Deficit may have difficulty organizing their notes logically so that they can be used for studying later on. They may need additional assistance to learn how to take notes in the first place, but can become quite adept at this task after training. Finally, note-taking may actually help some children with Associative Deficit to understand the information presented. By putting what is heard (but not necessarily completely understood at the time) into writing, then reading their notes later, these children often benefit from the dual-modality augmentation that note-taking provides.

Allowing the child to obtain notes from another student or even from the teacher, or providing a note-taker hired for the purpose, should be considered for some children with APD in middle school, high school, or college. But this decision, like all others regarding management of APD, should be made on the basis of the individual child's auditory difficulties. If the need to take notes is detracting from the student's ability to learn the key information presented in class, a note-taker may be needed.

- **Repeat *or* rephrase information, when appropriate.** On almost every central auditory assessment report that I see, the section on recommendations includes the following sentence: "The teacher should repeat or rephrase information." What is not always understood is that repetition is quite different from rephrasing. Whether repetition or rephrasing is appropriate depends entirely on the type of APD.

  By definition, repetition means that the speaker presents the message again using precisely the same language used the first time. Rephrasing, on the other hand, means to say the same thing in a different way, using different terminology or shorter, clearer language.

  The child with Auditory Decoding Deficit often benefits from direct repetition. He is able to fill in those portions of the message that were missed the first time around. If information is rephrased, however, this child now has an entirely new message to decode, with new missing pieces to figure out. Therefore, repetition is a more effective strategy for children with Auditory Decoding Deficit.

  In contrast, repetition is rarely effective for the child with Associative Deficit. Indeed, you can repeat a message over and over, but if it was not understood the first time, it will probably not be understood the second, fourth, or tenth time. Instead, rephrasing using smaller linguistic units (or chunks of information) and avoiding complex sentence forms (such as passive voice) is much more beneficial for the child with Associative Deficit. Similarly, children with Output-Organization Deficit will do better with smaller units of information, especially if they are allowed to act on each unit before the next is presented.

Children with Prosodic Deficit may benefit from either repetition or rephrasing, but only if key words in the message are emphasized strongly. Likewise, either strategy may be beneficial for children with Integration Deficit, as long as the information is presented clearly and other distractions—such as visual or tactile cues—are kept to a minimum.

This is an excellent example of why preprinted lists of suggestions for "all" children with APD should be avoided and management suggestions should be individualized for each child. Even a suggestion as seemingly innocuous as "repeat or rephrase information" can be implemented inappropriately unless the specific nature of the auditory deficit is taken into account.

- **Make *appropriate* use of visual cues and hands-on demonstrations.** When a child has any type of hearing or listening difficulty, it is usually helpful if the information presented verbally is augmented by visual cues and hands-on, tactile demonstrations—what we call multimodality cues. This allows the child to obtain input through those modalities that are stronger and adds to the auditory information so that the whole message can be understood. Even children with no type of disorder at all benefit from actually seeing and touching what is being discussed. That's why employing multimodality cues is one of the most common recommendations made for children with APD.

There is, however, an exception to this rule. Many children with Integration Deficit have, by definition, difficulty integrating multimodality cues. When provided with visual, tactile, and auditory information all at once, these children may become more confused than they would have been if the information had been presented through only one modality. I have often heard frustrated teachers say, "The more I try to help her, the worse she does!" When I hear this, I often suspect that the child is being bombarded with information through a variety of modalities and is simply incapable of integrating all of that information into one, clear message.

Children with Integration Deficit often do far better when information is presented sequentially; that is, when the message is first delivered verbally, *then* a picture of the topic is introduced, and *then* tactile cues (such as touching the actual object) are added. For example, during teaching of early math skills, numbers and manipulables (objects to be counted or added together, such as blocks or apples) are often used to convey basic number concepts. For the child with Integration Deficit, saying the numbers and operation ("1 plus 2"), *then* seeing the written numbers on the page, and *then* watching as the blocks are moved around to represent both the numbers and the mathematical operation will probably be far more effective than doing all three of these simultaneously. The child with Integration Deficit may become confused and attempt to focus on one item at a time (the blocks *or* the numbers on the page). As a result, she will miss the overall message entirely. When central auditory testing indicates that a child has Integration Deficit, I always recommend that she be monitored carefully to see if multimodality cues result in confusion or clarification.

Finally, the use of multimodality cuing is only effective if the visual or tactile cues match the information being presented verbally. For example, if the teacher is presenting a unit on transportation and is discussing trains, a picture of a truck would be inappropriate, even though a truck falls into the general transportation category. Similarly, if an object is being passed around the classroom, the teacher should not move on to another topic while the children are still focused on the object at hand. Therefore, when discussing outer space during science class, the teacher should let all of the students see and feel the moon rock before beginning to talk about satellites or lunar craters.

- **Preteach new information and vocabulary.** This can be an appropriate strategy for most children with APD and is often helpful even for students with no disorder. In fact, I frequently employ this method in my own graduate-level college courses. Before a new topic is introduced in class, key vocabulary and critical concepts can be presented in writing (or taught by a tutor) so that the student is already somewhat familiar with the words and ideas that will be presented. For example, the child with Auditory Decoding Deficit has problems filling in the missing pieces—or achieving closure—on some words even when they are familiar. Imagine the difficulty a child with this type of deficit would have when attempting to fill in the missing portions of a word he or she has never heard before. Provided the words in advance, the child will be ready for them during the classroom lecture and will be more likely to hear and understand them when they are spoken. Having students read the pertinent chapter in their textbook, familiarize themselves with new vocabulary, and learn basic concepts before the classroom lecture is an excellent way to enhance comprehension of new information for all students, from elementary school through college.

THINKING OUTSIDE THE BOX:
ENVIRONMENTAL MODIFICATIONS AT WORK

APD in a working adult presents a unique set of challenges. An adult with APD does not have the same level of support afforded children at school. Furthermore, although the adult with a disability is guaranteed some rights, he or she is not guaranteed, by law, the job itself. The person with APD must find ways to meet job expectations despite the APD. This is a minor concern for some adults with APD, but a major impediment for others. A computer programmer may find that APD does not affect his ability to perform his job, while a teacher, receptionist, or stockbroker may find APD debilitating. Management of APD in adults, as in children, should take into account the particular needs, type of deficit, and task-related demands of the person with the disorder.

Finding Alternative Ways to Perform I once worked with a dental hygienist with APD. Genny performed all of her job duties just fine, unless the dentist was filling a tooth. Then, the noise of the drill, combined with her difficulties hearing in noise, made Genny virtually unable to understand any directions the dentist gave.

Genny didn't know that she had an auditory processing deficit. All she knew was that she had occasional hearing difficulties, which hadn't bothered her much during her training to become a dental hygienist. Her teachers and the training dentists with whom she had worked had made good use of visual cues (demonstrating, pointing to the desired instruments) and approached each dental patient step by step with the same basic procedure. Genny had always known what to expect and had done quite well in both her academic classes and in her clinical practicum.

The dentist with whom Genny was working now, however, did not approach his craft in such a methodical manner. Genny never quite knew which instrument he was going to ask for or what he was likely to do next. In addition, he had a beard and a mustache, which limited Genny's ability to read his lips when he was talking. Finally, he issued commands in a rapid, terse manner and sighed in exasperation when Genny asked him to repeat what he had said. Often, he would fix her with a glare and get the requested instrument himself. By the time I first saw Genny, the dentist had become so frustrated with her that she had been relegated to answering the phone in the dental office—which, given her auditory difficulties, was not much better.

Genny had come to our clinic for an audiological evaluation because she had begun to wonder if a hearing loss was to blame for her difficulties, even though she had always passed hearing screenings during school. Her hearing acuity was entirely normal, but further testing confirmed the presence of an Auditory Decoding Deficit type of APD. Based on Genny's history, I suspect that her disorder had been present most, if not all, of her life.

To make accommodations that would assist Genny in doing the job she had been hired to do, we decided to include Genny's employer in our management plan. Although Genny was initially reluctant to approach him about this, I explained that it would be difficult, if not impossible, to implement changes in the workplace if the one person with whom she worked most often was not on board.

Genny thought her boss was short-tempered and grumpy, but to her surprise, he actually proved cooperative once the nature of her disorder was explained. "Hmmph. Well, that explains a lot," he said. "Now, what do we do about this damn thing?"

The first thing we did was to fit Genny with an FM system—an assistive listening device in which the dentist wore a small lapel microphone and Genny wore a receiver that delivered his voice directly into her ears. The system works on FM radio waves, so no wires connected the two. They could move about the room freely without restriction. Even when Genny was in another room, she could still hear and understand the dentist's voice. And she could hear everything he said clearly—even when he was drilling.

The dentist also began to explain his procedures to Genny more clearly—a strategy akin to preteaching. As it turned out, he had been following specific, step-by-step procedures. They were just different from what Genny had come to expect during training. And he had a different procedure for different types of patients. Once Genny understood his methods, and the rationale behind them, she was better able to anticipate his needs.

We also worked on Genny's communication needs in general: the need for the dentist to slow down a bit and face her when speaking to her, the need to avoid a lot of background noise (or to use the FM system) when issuing directions or giving information, and the need for the two of them to work together in the communicative effort.

Finally, we helped Genny take responsibility for her own listening success. Prior to this, she had been timid and afraid to speak up when she didn't hear something that was said, particularly because this was her first "real" job, and she was nervous about others' perceptions of her. After the dentist groused, "Well, you should have *told* me you couldn't hear me," Genny felt much more comfortable letting him know when she didn't understand. Ultimately, Genny realized that the final responsibility for informing others about her needs and ensuring that she could hear and understand rested on her own shoulders.

Today, Genny is able to do the job she had been trained for. She still works for the same dentist, and now, when he grouses at her, she grouses right back. They have come to a mutual understanding and have a close working relationship. Genny loves her chosen career.

When a working adult has APD that interferes with her ability to perform a chosen job, it is important to identify alternative ways to do the job. In Genny's case, the solutions were relatively simple and the outcome completely favorable. This is not always the case. In some situations, no solution can be arrived at, and a change in job setting or career may be the only choice. However, before making a dramatic decision involving a job or career change, every attempt should be made to resolve the difficulties in the current job setting. Some steps that can be helpful follow.

1. Analyze the environment. What is it about the job setting that, when coupled with the presence of APD, makes it so difficult to perform? Is there too much noise? Would an assistive listening device be helpful? Are certain coworkers easier to hear and understand than others? If so, what are they doing that others are not? Perhaps they speak more clearly or slowly. Perhaps they make sure their faces can be seen while talking. Perhaps they use clear, concise language. In any case, identify what works (and what doesn't) and make suggestions accordingly as to how supervisors and coworkers can best communicate.

2. Involve employers, supervisors, and coworkers in the management effort. An adult with APD needs to overcome his natural tendency to hide the disorder. He must be forthright regarding the nature of the disorder and the ways in which others can assist.

3. If hearing and understanding during staff meetings is difficult, consider some type of assistive listening or amplification device during these meetings. Alternatively, request minutes of each meeting so that information can be reviewed later. A written agenda given out before the meeting may also help orient an adult with APD to the topics that will be discussed.

4. If employers or others often deliver rapid-fire, complex instructions involving several steps, request that the information be provided in a written memo to verify that each step is clearly understood.

5. When in doubt, ask. Don't be afraid to request repetition or clarification when you don't understand. If you feel uncomfortable asking your supervisor or employer (or if such a move is simply

impractical), ask a well-informed coworker to go over the information and clarify any questions.

6. If an employer or coworker begins an important conversation at an inappropriate time—for example, while walking through a crowded hallway, during lunch in the cafeteria, or during another task—gently suggest that the conversation be moved to another location or scheduled for another time that would be more conducive to listening.

7. If background noise makes talking on the phone difficult, consider plugging the ear that is not being used or requesting that calls be rerouted to another, less noisy room.

8. Resist the urge to attribute all difficulties in the workplace to APD. Remember that many people without any type of disorder have difficulties with supervisors or coworkers. Try to determine which problems can be directly related to the auditory deficit.

9. Similarly, do not use APD as an excuse not to perform a job adequately. If completing assigned job duties is not possible even with accommodations, perhaps a change in job setting should be considered.

Knowing Your Legal Rights Under the provisions of the Americans with Disabilities Act (ADA), an employer cannot discriminate against an employee on the basis of a disability. If a person with a disability needs accommodations to perform his or her job, the employer is lawfully required to implement those accommodations. An employee in a wheelchair who is completely capable of performing a given job if she could just get up the three steps into the office has the legal right to request that a wheelchair ramp or other means of access be supplied. Similarly, the person with diagnosed APD has the right to request reasonable accommodations.

An important distinction should be made here: there is a difference between needing accommodations because of a disability to do the job appropriately and being unable to do the job at all. There is also a difference between being afforded legal job rights as a person with a disability and being hired *because* of the disability. Under ADA, a *qualified* person cannot be discriminated against because of a disability. However, ADA does not guarantee the job itself. If a disability renders a person unable to perform in a given career, that person is not entitled by law to be hired. Some jobs—bus driver, pilot, and radio dispatcher, for example—require a certain level of visual and auditory acuity before the person can even be hired. The key point is that the person should be able to complete the job duties once accommodations are in place.

Federal law affords every school-aged child a free and appropriate education. Federal law does not afford every adult a job. It does, however, ensure that a person cannot be discriminated against on the basis of a disability. If you feel that you have been passed over for promotion, treated unfairly in the workplace, or not hired at all solely because of a disability (and not because of lack of education, skills, or similar performance-related problems), you should seek legal aid.

Taking Responsibility in the Workplace The responsibility for hearing, understanding, and following through on directions and information at work rests firmly on the shoulders of the employee. At school, a multidisciplinary team looks after the child with a disability and helps ensure that she learns. But no one watches over the adult with APD to make sure she does her job. In schools, team meetings are convened to make sure that everyone knows about the child's disorder and how to best meet the child's needs. At work, there is no team, no behind-the-scenes group of people whose job is to develop and implement a plan to meet the needs of the adult with APD. And no one informs significant coworkers, supervisors, and others about the nature of the APD and how to communicate with the person who has it. No one, that is, except the adult with APD.

If you are a working adult with APD, you must communicate your needs. You should also provide your employer written documentation of your disorder from your audiologist, along with suggestions for management, for placement in your personnel file. But don't approach the situation like an offensive linebacker barreling through the opponent's team. Couching your needs in the form of demands, telling the employer what he *must* do, and forcefully reminding him that federal law states that reasonable accommodations must be made will only alienate him. On the other hand, you should not be overly apologetic about your disorder, either.

You should explain the nature of your disorder matter-of-factly, describe how it affects your communication abilities (giving examples whenever possible), and present general ideas regarding the types of accommodations that are helpful. You should then enlist the employer as a team player in devising means specific to your workplace that can accommodate your needs effectively and efficiently. At all times, you should endeavor to make your recommendations reasonable for your specific job setting, and you should explain why each accommodation is necessary. For example, providing written minutes and memos or an assistive listening device might be considered a reasonable accommodation. Provision of a personal secretary or aide to monitor your performance, keep you on target, manage your projects, and take on some of your tasks would not.

Finally, you should always keep the job requirements themselves at the forefront of the conversation so that the employer gets the clear message that you are having this conversation so that you can be a better employee. You must always remember that, no matter how personable and caring an employer may be, his primary concern is whether your job will be done to specifications, not your personal happiness or satisfaction. You must be able to assure your employer that this is your primary concern, as well.

A disorder or disability should never be used as an excuse for performing a job poorly. If you are unable to perform your job because of your disorder, even with appropriate and reasonable accommodations in place, you and your employer should revisit the issue and determine whether different management approaches might be more effective. However, if you are still unable to perform after all options have been exhausted, it may be time to look for another job that does not involve the same communicative or auditory demands. We all have areas of relative strength and weakness, skills that we excel at and tasks that we find quite difficult. When we match our job or career decisions with our strengths and skills, it makes for a much happier and satisfying work experience for all concerned.

WHERE THEY HAVE TO TAKE YOU IN: ENVIRONMENTAL MODIFICATIONS AT HOME

When a person has a disability, the impact on the family can be even more devastating than on academics or work. Coping with and compensating for APD at school or work can be exhausting. Yet, many people with APD are far more successful at dealing with their difficulties when in a structured work or school environment or in public. At home, no one wants to work that hard. Home is a place for putting your feet up, letting your hair down, and being yourself. Even people who are adept at compensating for APD outside the home may find themselves having great difficulty communicating at the end of the day. Frustrations that were suppressed at school or work may be transferred to family members at home. Sheer exhaustion may make for a grumpy, tearful child; a sullen, withdrawn teenager; or an angry adult. Many of us have these tendencies after a hard day at work or school, but they may be much more pronounced in the person with APD.

Nevertheless, one has responsibilities at home. There are chores to be done, supper to be prepared, dishes to be washed. There is the need for conversation among family members. It can be a source of endless frustration when listening skills perfected at school or work are not employed at home. The unique nature of home and family dynamics requires different management approaches and considerations from those that are reasonable in other settings. A delicate balance must be struck between allowing the person with APD to take a break from it all and seeing that he meets expectations and responsibilities at home.

The Need for Acceptance There is perhaps no place in the world where acceptance is more needed, and more expected, than at home among family and loved ones. Everyone needs to be accepted for who he or she is, bad habits and all. A person with APD must feel loved despite the disorder. Sometimes, however, parents, spouse, and others may unintentionally send the message that the person with APD is a burden, unloved and unappreciated.

Consider the following common scenario: Jimmy, a fourth-grader with APD, comes home from school on a Friday afternoon. He is elated that he passed his spelling test that day and proudly presents a note from the teacher that reads, "Jimmy is listening and following directions much better in the classroom and on the playground. He is working very hard to be a good listener and we think that the suggestions made at his IEP meeting are really having an excellent impact on his ability to understand and complete his schoolwork. He earned a 95% on his spelling test today and it is very apparent that Jimmy studied this week. We are quite proud of him!"

Jimmy's mother smiles and hugs him, telling him that she, too, is proud. She fixes him a snack and he goes into the family room to watch television for a while. He is looking forward to the weekend fishing trip that his father has promised him if he passed his spelling exam.

An hour later, Jimmy's mother calls from the kitchen, "That's enough television for now. Your father will be home soon, so I'd like you to set the table. Oh, and you need to move your backpack and coat away from the front door so he doesn't trip over them when he comes in. Make sure you put knives out; we're having steak."

Jimmy slowly picks up his backpack and coat and tosses them onto the floor in front of the hall closet, his eyes never leaving the television screen. Task completed, he curls up on the sofa once again.

Fifteen minutes later, his mother calls again from the kitchen: "Jimmy? Where are you? I told you to set the table! Turn that television off now!"

Reluctantly, Jimmy turns off the set and makes his way into the kitchen. Carefully, he places three sets of plates, glasses, napkins, and forks onto the table. As he is helping his mother put the finishing touches on the dinner preparation, Jimmy's father enters the front door with jacket and briefcase in hand, makes his way to the closet, and promptly trips over Jimmy's backpack and coat.

"Jimmy!" he bellows. "Come get your stuff right now and put it away where it belongs!"

"I told you to put that away so your father wouldn't trip over it," Jimmy's mother scolds. "Get in there right now and do what I told you!"

A few minutes later, Jimmy and his parents sit down for dinner. Excitedly, Jimmy tells his father about his spelling test. "I got an A! And the teacher wrote a note and said I was listening real good! So that means we'll go fishing this weekend, right?"

His mother interrupts him: "Jimmy, where are the knives?"

"The what?"

"The steak knives. I told you we're having steak and to put knives on the table."

"I didn't hear you."

Exasperated, his mother shakes her head. "No, you just weren't listening. You were too busy watching television. You *never* listen."

"But my teacher says I'm a good listener now."

"Maybe at school, but not here. I'm your mother. Don't I deserve the same respect you give your teacher? Why can't you listen to me the way you listen to her? You didn't hear me because the television was just too important."

"Until you start following directions at home and listening to your mother, there'll be no more TV for you," says Jimmy's father sternly. "Your mother and I are sick and tired of the way you ignore us. You come home with notes talking about how great you're doing in school, but *we* sure don't see any of that great stuff. You still can't listen to your own mother when she tells you to do something as simple as put knives on the table. I'll tell you, things are gonna change around here, buddy, right now. And you're not setting one foot outside of this house until they do!"

"What about the fishing trip?" Jimmy whispers.

"You can forget about that until you start pulling your own weight in this family and doing what you're told. Now, go to your room and think about it. Your mother and I want to eat in peace."

Scenarios such as this one are not entirely uncommon in households with young children. But when a child has APD, they occur much more frequently and can be even more frustrating for everyone. In some ways, Jimmy was behaving like a typical kid on a Friday afternoon: lounging in front of the television and "ignoring" his mother. On the other hand, that Jimmy's mother issued her commands from the kitchen without first making sure that she had obtained his attention and could be heard clearly may have set Jimmy up for failure. Adding to his parents' frustration is the glowing report from Jimmy's teacher concerning his much improved listening skills at school, which seems to be in stark contrast to the current home situation. What began as something to be proud of (improvement in listening at school) has become a point of contention and unfavorable comparison when the same good listening skills were not displayed at home. Finally, Jimmy's hard-earned reward—the fishing trip—was revoked because of an incident that was unrelated to the behavior that had earned him the reward in the first place: his good grade on the spelling exam.

Parents get frustrated with children—that is a fact of life. Children don't always listen—that, too, is a fact of life. But when a child has APD and a great deal of attention has been given to listening skills, this typical, common argument can evolve into something much more significant and serious. Jimmy may have come away with the conviction that his parents only love the "good-listener Jimmy" and not the "bad-listener Jimmy." In addition, the good-listener Jimmy must be present at all times, at home and at school, for his parents to truly accept and love him. Good listening at school doesn't count, no matter how much effort he exerts or how successful he is. If it did, the wonderful note from his teacher and the A on his spelling test would not have been forgotten just because of the missing steak knives. But Jimmy knows he can't be a good listener all the time. No child can, especially a child with an auditory processing deficit. Therefore, Jimmy may well be left with the feeling that he will never be completely acceptable to his parents, no matter how hard he tries.

This type of situation occurs not only between parents and children. It is perhaps even more common between spouses. Even when an APD is known to and understood by both parties, there will inevitably be times when frustration or anger is expressed because of something that wasn't heard or understood. Comments made in the heat of anger, such as "I can't stand it anymore. I'm so tired of having to tell you things over and over again before you hear me" may be taken as "I don't love you anymore" by the person with APD.

To avoid this type of misconception and to help ensure that the person with APD feels accepted in spite of his disorder, bear in mind—and, where possible, act upon—the following tips:

1. Blame the disorder, not the person. Instead of saying, "I am so angry at *you* because you never listen to me," express your anger at the disorder itself. This allows the person with APD to agree and say, "Yeah, this thing is frustrating for me, too." Battle the common enemy of APD. Don't battle each other.

2. Separate the person from the disorder. APD does not define a person; however, the incredible amount of attention devoted to

diagnosing and managing APD can make someone feel as if nothing else about her is important. Try to focus equally on good skills, not just on the listening-related negative behaviors. Make it clear that disliking APD is not the same as disliking the person with APD.

3. Let the punishment fit the crime. Try to avoid the roller coaster of praising the person with APD for good listening one minute, then rejecting him for poor listening the next. If a child does something that is unacceptable, address *that* behavior accordingly. Do not take away a reward previously earned for good behavior.

4. Avoid saying "You never . . ." When you are frustrated, it may be difficult to remember that the person with APD is trying and does exhibit good listening skills some of the time. Make sure to acknowledge that good listening behaviors do occur. "You never . . ." may eventually become a self-fulfilling prophecy. After all, if previous successes are continually negated in this manner, why try to succeed at all? Along these same lines, keep the discussion to the situation at hand and do not bring up past miscommunications. Listing previous failures only serves to further the feeling that the person is unacceptable, unloved, and a failure.

5. Avoid comparing listening environments. Remember that most people with APD will perform better when in a structured situation such as at school or work. They need to feel free to relax and be themselves at home. Don't expect the same type of focused effort at home as at work or school.

6. Analyze problem situations and talk about them. What was it that led to the misunderstanding? What was due to inattention or behavior, and what was due to the disorder?

7. Avoid overemphasizing auditory behavior. Everyone misunderstands or mishears at times. Not every situation requires an in-

depth analysis or full-blown confrontation. Sometimes, it is more important just to clarify the message, let go, and move on. Try not to turn every miscommunication into an extended diatribe on APD.

Generalization of Skills to the Home Environment Despite the need for acceptance in the home, it is still important for the person with APD to put forth an effort. Skills implemented in the more structured environments of school or work should, to some degree, be carried over to the home. Only then will chores, instructions, rules, and other communications be understood and acted upon. The child or adult with APD is not off the hook completely once he or she walks through the front door. The unstructured home environment may make this generalization of skills difficult, so different strategies will be needed at home.

The entire family should help come up with ideas on how to manage APD at home. Modifications and communication strategies that have been found to be effective in school or at work can be adapted for the home. Remember, though, that the ultimate goal of home management of APD is to facilitate communication while, at the same time, maintaining the warm, friendly, accepting atmosphere of safety and family. Therefore, the home environment shouldn't be too structured or it will seem less like a place to escape to at the end of the day and more like just another job or school setting.

Following are some tips that may help:

1. Family members should agree on *when* and *where* important information will be conveyed. It is difficult for anyone to hear and understand someone talking when the television is blaring and the baby is crying. It is even more difficult for a person with APD. Simply stepping into another room or turning off the television and gaining the person's visual attention can go a long way toward preventing misunderstandings.

2. In spy movies, key characters get together and synchronize their watches before a caper. Football players gather in the locker room and go over game plans before the big game. These types of activities can be very useful when a family member has APD. Set a time to get together and make plans, assign chores, and handle important business. This may be a daily or weekly event, depending on the circumstances. Write everything down on a notepad or, even better, a reusable write-on/wipe-off board. As decisions are made, list who is responsible for what and the expected timeline. The board then serves several functions: it clarifies any potential misunderstandings, serves as a visual reminder of expectations and responsibilities, and provides a convenient means of follow-up.

3. Remember, different types of APD require different types of communication strategies.

   a. If someone in your family has Auditory Decoding Deficit, pay special attention to the acoustic environment. Make sure that you have visual attention before speaking, and whenever you can, make sure you demonstrate visually what is expected. If a message is not heard or understood, repeat it or write it down. Do not try to carry on a conversation when someone is vacuuming, washing dishes, or engaged in another activity that involves competing noise.

   b. If the family member has a Prosodic Deficit, pay special attention to *how* you say things and make sure to explain your intentions whenever possible. Don't hint. Spell out your meaning. To avoid miscommunications, misunderstandings, and hurt feelings, avoid being too subtle or abstract. Don't use long, complicated sentences in which the main point is hidden in a lot of unnecessary language. Pay special attention to saying (and explaining, when needed) precisely what you mean. Remember, too, that sarcasm, humor, and subtle hints may go unnoticed or be misinterpreted by someone with Prosodic Deficit.

c. For children or adults with Interhemispheric Deficit, remember that visual or tactile distractions may be just as destructive to comprehension as auditory distractions. Try not to carry on important conversations while engaged in distracting activities such as putting groceries away or exercising together or while the person is writing or doing homework. In addition, make sure that you give critical information *via one modality at a time*. For example, if you are helping a child build a model airplane, don't try to explain the next step while, at the same time, pointing to the instruction sheet and holding the pieces together as a demonstration. Read the instruction together first, *then* explain it (if necessary), and *then* demonstrate how the pieces should fit together.

d. For family members, especially children, with more language-based or executive-function-based auditory deficits such as Associative or Output-Organization Deficit, remember to keep your communications simple. If several steps are to be completed or several chores done, you may need to provide them one at a time and allow the child to complete each one before presenting the next. To avoid needing to call the child again and again for each chore, which is often frustrating for everyone, you might want to tell him, "Check back when you're done for your next job." If you make that a general rule, you won't continually need to regain the child's attention for each and every step. If the child does not understand the message, don't just repeat it. Instead, rephrase using simpler language. Finally, as with many other types of APD, writing down the steps, chores, or expectations sequentially and posting them where the child can refer to them will save time and energy for everyone.

4. Always remember that people with APD may not know when they aren't hearing or understanding correctly. Although they may sometimes ask for clarification (or respond with a look of confusion), don't count on it. Indeed, children or adults with APD often complete a task proudly, only to find that what they *thought* they were supposed to do was inaccurate. Try not to punish or reject them for this. Instead, realize that they may have honestly thought that they were doing the right thing. Ask the person to retell you what you've said and/or monitor the behavior (at least initially) to see that she is on task. Finally, never discourage someone from asking for repetitions by saying, "Again? Weren't you listening?" You want them to request repetition or clarification when something is not heard or understood. If requests for repetition occur far too frequently, examine how you are communicating to determine how you can convey the message more clearly in the first place.

5. Collaborate with family members with APD to determine what communication modifications work best. Ask directly how best to communicate. They may say, "I understand best when you . . ." or "I have a hard time hearing or understanding you when . . ." Once those criteria are identified, make every effort to abide by them. For example, my husband has told me clearly over and over that he cannot hear me when there is noise (such as water running) nearby. He has requested that I wait until he turns the water off before talking to him. I don't always remember to honor his request, but when I don't, I try to accept the responsibility for any miscommunications that occur during those times. I knew the rules. I broke them. It's no one's fault but my own.

6. Finally, and most importantly, keep a sense of humor. The miscommunications that accompany APD can be incredibly frustrating. But they can also be terribly funny at times, too. A mother once told me a story about her son, who had an Auditory

Decoding Deficit type of APD. It was a lovely summer day. Many of the neighbors were out in their yards barbecuing or just sitting and enjoying the soft breeze. This mother had instructed her son to go outside and play with their new puppy while she finished putting away the laundry. A few minutes later, she heard her sweet little boy yelling a particularly profane word at the top of his lungs, over and over. She ran to the back door, threw it open, and was excruciatingly aware of the shocked looks on the neighbors' faces as she yelled to her son, "Stop that and come here, right now!" Fully prepared to give him a thorough tongue-lashing, she asked him what in the world he thought he was doing and who had taught him that horrible language. He replied, "Mr. Carver, next door. He was watching Alfie jump all over me and he said that I should tell him to shit. I tried, but he just wouldn't listen. Maybe he has APD, too?"

What About Me? Siblings of Children with APD I grew up with a deaf brother. I am intimately aware of what it is like to be a "normal" sibling of a child with a disability. I have also spoken to adults and children from all over the world who have been in similar situations, and many common themes have appeared in our communications. When a child has a disorder such as APD, sometimes so much time and money and effort are spent on addressing the disorder that little is left over for the other, nondisordered siblings. The nondisordered sibling is likely to see the disabled brother or sister as getting more attention, more breaks, more rewards, more everything. Whether these feelings are founded in fact or not, this can lead to feelings of resentment, abandonment, and self-doubt on the part of the nondisordered brother or sister, feelings that can persist even into adulthood.

Many of these feelings arise from normal sibling rivalry that plagues every family with more than one child. Who among us with children has not heard, "He gets to do everything, and I don't get to do *anything!*" But when a brother or sister has a disability, there may be very real bases for the normal siblings' feelings and perceptions. Often, and completely unintentionally, parents *do* give the child with a disorder more applause for accomplishments, more leeway to break rules, and certainly more time together, especially in those early years when the evaluations and therapy sessions seem endless. Although they would be horrified to realize it, these parents may—without meaning to—be sending subtle signals to their nondisordered children that they are not as important as the disordered son or daughter. Even parents who try hard to treat each of their children equally may fall into this trap. They may be completely unaware of how their nondisordered children are feeling. In contrast, other parents may be acutely aware that they are focusing much more on the child with a disorder and express feelings of guilt, frustration, and helplessness at trying to manage a family while, at the same time, engaging in activities that are necessary to diagnose and address one child's disorder. Finally, many parents may feel the need to justify vehemently, albeit regretfully, the inequality of attention given to the children in the family because one child's disorder necessitates activities that are just not required for the other children. These parents may react quite defensively to any mention of possible adverse effects on the nondisordered children.

Some siblings of children with disorders become overachievers, trying hard to do everything to gain positive attention for their actions, including serving as caretakers for their disordered brothers or sisters. Others may take the opposite road and seek attention through negative behaviors that force the parents to acknowledge them. Some complain of health, hearing, vision, or learning problems of their own so that they, too, can qualify for the same treatment they feel their brothers or sisters are getting. And many siblings of children with disorders alternate among all three of these patterns, trying to see which works best.

Just as many parents may not always be aware of their own subtle behaviors, many siblings of disordered children are not consciously aware of the motivations and emotions that give rise to their own actions. Indeed, they may go through their entire lifetimes never openly acknowledging—either to themselves or to others—their feelings of jealousy and resentment. They may even vehemently deny that they have ever experienced any such feelings at all. Their denial often arises from deep-seated feelings of guilt. After all, *they* don't have a disorder. They should feel lucky. What type of terrible person would be jealous of a family member who is suffering from a disability?

Nevertheless, research into siblings of disordered children, an area that has only recently begun to receive increasing attention in the literature, shows clearly that a sibling of a disordered child rarely goes through childhood without feeling any of these emotions. And for the vast majority, these feelings are far more than fleeting. Instead, they are often pervasive and have a lasting, lifetime impact on self-perception and behavior.

Therefore, as we consider managing APD in the home, we must consider the needs of the nondisordered siblings. Here are some suggestions that help to lessen the emotional impact of a child's being the "other kid."

1. Even the playing field and applaud achievements equally. Try to avoid setting different levels of expectation for children in the same family. For example, if a young boy with APD earns a B in reading after much hard work, it is entirely appropriate to hug him and exclaim gleefully over his success. But remember to provide his sister or brother with the same enthusiastic response for the same result, even if he or she is capable of A work. It is very difficult for a nondisordered child to understand why a sibling's B might be met with the response "Great job!" whereas his or her B is met with "You could have done a little better." This is true even if the nondisordered sibling is capable of performing at a higher level. Although parents may fear that this approach will lead the nondisordered child to be satisfied with mediocre per-

formance and will result in a lack of motivation to aspire to anything greater, the opposite is true. Children who are reinforced
in this way often respond with even greater effort so that their
parents will be even more proud of them. And in the process,
they are continually reminded that their parents love them and
are proud of them no matter what.

2. Provide negative reinforcements (or punishment) equally. Set
the same standards of behavior for all children in the family. Although some disorders prevent a child from adhering to normal
behavioral expectations, APD is not one of them. Children with
APD should not get away with behaviors that would be unacceptable for their siblings.

3. Never, ever, say or even imply that the nondisordered sibling's
achievements required less effort than those of the child with
APD. I was once told of a boy with a hearing disorder who came
home from school with B's and a few A's on his report card. The
boy was proud of his achievements, as he should have been.
When his nondisordered sister pointed out (admittedly, somewhat imperiously) that *she* had earned straight A's, the parents responded, "Yes, but that comes easy for you." Clearly the parents'
primary motivation was to avoid making the boy with APD feel
inferior for his grades in comparison to his sister's. However, the
unintentional result was that the sister was made to feel that her
accomplishments didn't matter, that her own hard work and effort was completely dismissed.

4. Explain the nature of APD to other children in the family so that
they can understand the disorder and how it affects learning,
language, and communication. But be careful not to suggest that
the child is entitled to special consideration in the family because
of the disorder. This may lead the nondisordered siblings to wish
for a disorder themselves, so that they will also earn such special

treatment. It may even lead to malingering behaviors in which the sibling begins to behave as if he or she does, indeed, have some sort of disorder. Discuss ways to foster communication with the child with APD, and don't forget to ask the nondisordered sibling about his or her own needs. For example, if the child with APD needs instructions to be presented one step at a time or written down, ask the sibling if he or she would like to get instructions in the same manner. Often, the nondisordered brother or sister will decline, but will be happy that his or her needs were considered and will be less likely to resent the child with APD for special accommodations.

5. Many parents think that they can make nondisordered children feel important and needed if they are enlisted to help the child with APD. Statements such as "You know, you're such a good reader, you can help Johnny with his reading and spelling" are commonplace in families that have children with APD. However, parents should be careful not to force a sibling into a caretaker role. This can result in significant resistance and resentment, especially if the nondisordered sibling is younger than the child with APD. Moreover, it can set up a dependent relationship between siblings that persists into adulthood, with the person with APD continually relying on his or her sibling to assist with difficult tasks. This type of responsibility should be delegated only when the nondisordered brother or sister first expresses interest—either verbally or through his or her behavior—in taking on such a caretaker role. Even then, the nondisordered child should never be expected to continually put his or her own needs behind those of the sibling with APD. On the other hand, when the nondisordered sibling is older than the child with APD, he or she should be held to the normal big-sister or big-brother expectations of watching out for the littler kids that occur in any family with more than one child.

6. When frustrated or angry, parents often say things they regret later. In families in which one child has a disorder, parents may react to complaints or expressions of jealousy or unfair treatment from the nondisordered sibling by pointing out that he is "lucky" and should be grateful for the abilities that the child with APD does not have. Chances are the nondisordered sibling does not feel lucky or grateful at that moment. He probably feels unappreciated, overlooked, or ignored and feels guilty for those emotions. Acknowledge the child's feelings and give them validation rather than telling him that he shouldn't have them in the first place.

7. Strive to spend equal time with each child in the family. In today's fast-paced world, it sometimes seems impossible to do everything in twenty-four short hours a day. When a child with APD is being shuttled from evaluation to evaluation, or to and from therapy sessions, time is taken away from other family members. Explaining that assessments or therapy sessions don't exactly meet the criteria for quality one-on-one time with Mom or Dad is futile. The nondisordered sibling just cares about the amount of time (and therefore, attention) that is devoted to the child with APD. It is important for parents to schedule similar one-on-one time with the other children in the family, even though doing so may be difficult given everyone's hectic schedule. One way this can be accomplished is to have the nondisordered sibling accompany the parent and child with APD to therapy sessions. While the child with APD is in therapy, the other family members can sit in the waiting room and read a book together, play a game, discuss school activities, and spend true quality time together.

These are just a few tips for addressing the "What about me?" dilemma. We shouldn't, however, forget one other important family member who, likewise, may feel left out or ignored when a child has a disability. Every effort should be made to meet the needs of the nondisordered children in the family, but spouses have the same needs, too. The need for one-on-one quality time between spouses is often overlooked. Indeed, after each day spent trying to meet the needs of all children in the family as well as working a job and attending to all of life's other chores, it is most often the husband or wife who gets ignored. Parents need time away from the concerns of the world to focus just on each other.

TRAINING THE BRAIN: THERAPY ACTIVITIES FOR APD

Environmental modifications make information more accessible to the person with APD, but they do not remediate the disorder. The second component of any APD management program is direct therapy. I have often heard it said that APD cannot be "fixed" and that the best we can do is to teach methods of compensating for it and managing it in daily life. However, recent research into neuroplasticity—the ability of the brain to change, reorganize, and make new and stronger connections in response to the presence or absence of stimulation— clearly shows that auditory training can treat some cases of APD. We know, for example, that lack of stimulation can result in poor auditory processing skills and that these poor skills are accompanied by structural changes in the brain pathways dedicated to auditory processing. We also know that auditory training—therapy activities to develop listening skills—can, likewise, result in positive structural and functional changes of the central auditory pathways. Finally, we know that any type of auditory training must be frequent, intense, and challenging for it to have the greatest impact.

But how frequent? How intense? And specifically what types of auditory training are most effective? And for whom? The research into therapeutic efficacy for APD is in its infancy, and there is so much that we do not yet know. Even though direct therapy has been amazingly successful for some children and adults with APD, essentially "fixing" the disorder completely and restoring normal auditory processing function, this is not always the case. In fact, we more commonly see some improvement in auditory processing and related skills, but not a complete remediation of the problem. We can't predict how successful any therapy program will be for a specific child or adult. This is why we teach people with APD methods of compensating for the residual deficits that may remain even after therapy. Nevertheless, our ultimate goal is to ameliorate the disorder, and that is the focus of much of our current research in the field of APD. Right now, we have a lot of information and knowledge to help guide us in that quest, and more and more information is becoming available daily to help us streamline the process and make therapy more efficient and effective.

Matching the Therapy to the Disorder Treatment approaches should be directed toward the type of APD that a given child or adult has and those auditory areas that are causing a problem. Of course, the key to determining which specific therapy or treatment approach to use is having an accurate, complete diagnosis of the disorder and knowing how that disorder affects the person's learning, language, and communication.

Combining Resources Unlike diagnosis of APD, for which the audiologist is the only qualified professional, treatment of APD may be undertaken by a variety of professionals. In fact, it should be a multidisciplinary team approach.

Most children with APD are already receiving some type of therapy or assistance for associated difficulties with reading, spelling, language, or other academic or communication areas. When an APD is diagnosed, we need to address the auditory difficulties without ignoring these other important areas. We also want to avoid inundating the child with so much therapy that little time is left over for leisure.

Therapy for APD is most effective and efficient when we combine our resources. For example, the reading tutor or resource room reading specialist may include phonological and speech-sound discrimination training in his or her reading or spelling therapy program. In this way, time is saved and the auditory skills taught are directly related to the reading and spelling difficulties the child is having. Similarly, children receiving speech and language therapy often benefit from a combined approach including both auditory perception and spoken production goals. These approaches are particularly useful when the child is receiving direct special education services in the schools, because they promote learning across various areas and result in maximum overall benefit when resources are limited.

On the other hand, the research is clear that frequent, intense, and challenging auditory training and stimulation will result in the greatest amount of improvement in auditory skills. Therefore, specific auditory training to address deficit areas is important for many children and adults with APD. When the training requires special audiological equipment, the audiologist may provide these services. However, few audiologists specialize in treatment of APD. More commonly, it is the speech-language pathologist or other professional who will supervise and provide such therapy. It really doesn't matter which professional is providing the service as long as the therapy technique is appropriate for the individual's auditory deficit.

Issues of frequency and intensity are also important. Research has yet to uncover the minimum amount of time required to achieve maximum benefit from specific auditory training therapy; however, evidence suggests that maximum benefit requires a substantial commitment, usually forty-five to ninety minutes per day, five days per week, for several weeks. To expect this degree of commitment from school-based professionals, who may have hundreds of children in their caseloads, is clearly unreasonable. Moreover, if a child were to undergo this degree of therapy during the school day, he or she would miss many classes and would not learn the academic information that is the purpose of school. Finally, federal law does not require or even support the provision of this degree of therapy in schools. Therefore, intensive auditory training programs or services are usually provided through university or private clinics, and payment for such services is usually the parents' responsibility.

As to *when* such intensive training should occur, one common approach is to schedule daily training sessions after school or in the early evenings. When therapy sessions are scheduled twice per week or so, this approach is acceptable. However, when intense programs that require daily training for an extended time are implemented, we may overwhelm and exhaust the child, who already faces a challenging school day. I often suggest that children undergo time-intensive programs during summer vacation or when they can devote appropriate energy to the training while still having time left over for more enjoyable activities and rest.

In my experience, the most effective plan for treating APD incorporates auditory-based activities into existing learning- or language-related services, combined with more intensive auditory-specific training outside of school and when the danger of overload is at a minimum.

Types of Therapy Activities   There are so many different approaches to and techniques for auditory training that it is impossible to discuss all of them here. In addition, more and more techniques are being developed daily. Some approaches are commercially available and, thus, may be familiar to parents and others. On the other hand, many effective therapy approaches have been developed and are being implemented by individual clinicians but are not commercially available or well-known. These approaches take many different forms, but have one goal in common: to directly address the specific auditory deficit exhibited by the particular child or adult with APD.

Before we consider some categories of auditory training activities a little more closely, I should emphasize that choosing a program or technique requires professional guidance. We must rely on a physician to prescribe a certain medication to treat an illness. Similarly, the type of therapy "prescribed" for a person's APD is a decision best left up to trained professionals, who can take all of the information into account and arrive at an appropriate strategy. I should also emphasize that many reading, spelling, and learning programs have become popular for use with children who have learning difficulties due to APD. These are not, however, auditory training programs and should not be considered treatment programs for APD. Rather, they are often extremely beneficial in helping the child with APD, along with many others who do not have APD, learn to read, spell, or write. I myself have recommended some of these programs for many of my own patients. However, our discussion here will be confined to those categories of therapy activities that truly are auditory in nature.

- **Phonological awareness activities.** These activities focus on speech-sound processing and may include discriminating between speech sounds that are similar (e.g., *da* versus *ga*); discriminating between vowel sounds (e.g., *a* as in *cat* versus *e* as in *egg*); identifying speech sounds that occur in the beginning, middle, or end of words; segmenting words into their individual speech sounds (e.g., CAT = C . . . A . . . T); blending speech sounds into whole words (e.g., C . . . A . . . T = CAT); and similar activities. Often, the listening portion of these activities is combined with recognizing the associated written letters or words to facilitate reading and spelling skills and strengthen sound-symbol association abilities. The advent of computer-based programs for phonological awareness and speech-sound discrimination provides stimuli that sound much more similar than we could produce with our own voices while also engaging the child or adult with interesting visual graphics. As a result, phonological awareness skills can be sharpened even further. However, live-voice speech-sound training and sound-symbol association activities continue to be useful. These activities are most appropriate for those with speech-sound based APD, specifically Auditory Decoding Deficit.

- **Auditory closure Activities.** Activities that focus on using the context of the situation or conversation to fill in the missing pieces are appropriate for people with Auditory Decoding Deficit and others for whom auditory closure skills are a problem. With small children, we may use familiar nursery rhymes (e.g., "Twinkle, twinkle, little_____"). For older children and adults, we progress to sentences in which words are omitted (e.g., "Babe Ruth hit the____with the bat") and to words in which speech sounds are missing (e.g., "ba__ball"). Again, the advent of computer technology has allowed us to more cleanly edit out speech sounds in words; however, these activities can be performed live-voice, as well. Another form of auditory closure activity is training in speech-in-noise skills. Once the person has mastered a given activity in quiet listening situations, noise of varying levels is added to make the activity more challenging. These activities may also be useful for those with Associative Deficit to help them grasp the meaning of a message; however, therapy for this type of deficit usually focuses primarily on receptive language abilities rather than specific auditory skills.

- **Selective attention and localization activities.** Many people with APD have difficulty telling where a sound is coming from or with listening to one message while ignoring another, competing message. These people often benefit from specific training in dichotic listening. In this type of training, the listener's attention is directed toward the weaker ear. The sound levels of each ear are adjusted to make the listening activity more challenging as the person progresses. A related activity is to identify the source of a sound as being to the right or the left of the person, first in quiet and then in noise. As the person becomes better at this, the sound sources are brought closer and closer together. These activities require electronic equipment and/or audiologic sound booths. Some are computer-based and require stereo headphones. They are most appropriate for people with APD that affects hemispheric dominance, especially those with interhemispheric Integration Deficit.

- **Temporal patterning training.** Temporal patterning activities address rhythm and related skills. For the most part, these techniques are nonverbal and may involve clapping, tapping on the table, or similar activities. Linguistic stimuli such as words can be used; however, the focus here is not on the speech sounds themselves, but rather on the rhythm, stress, and pitch of the auditory stimuli over time. Activities may include imitating the rhythm of a series of claps that increase in complexity and length, identifying which clap (or tone or word) in a series is louder than the others, and identifying which tone in a series is higher or lower in pitch. Ultimately, focus can be placed on the imitation of the entire "acoustic contour," or of the rhythm, loudness, and pitch patterns of a stimulus simultaneously. These activities are appropriate for APD that affects the ability to perceive nonlinguistic changes in rhythm, stress, and pitch, such as Prosodic Deficit.

- **Prosody training.** People with Prosodic Deficit often require specific therapy for interpreting tone-of-voice cues and other nonlinguistic information. For example, telling the difference between surprise and anger sometimes requires interpretation of subtle voice and body cues. Questions, jokes, and sarcasm rely on recognition of subtle changes in tone of voice. For some words or sentences, the entire meaning can differ depending on where the stress is placed (e.g., *convict* versus con*vict;* "*You* can't go with me" versus "You can't go with *me*"). Fun activities such as role-playing and charades can make prosody training quite enjoyable. Finally, prosody training is most effective when both perception and production are worked on in tandem. That is, the focus should be on both understanding these subtle prosody cues as well as on *using* them in spoken language.

- **Interhemispheric exercises.** Activities that force the two halves of the brain to work together are often helpful for people with interhemispheric Integration Deficit. These activities can include music (especially piano or guitar) lessons, sensory integration activities, sports that require both hands or both feet (such as soccer), video games that require bimanual reactions, and so on. Dichotic listening training in which the person, using stereo headphones, listens to both ears simultaneously while adjusting the relative loudness levels between ears is also useful. Many of these activities are particularly suited for home-based therapy and can involve the entire family. Some of these activities may also be indicated for those with Output-Organization Deficit; however, therapy for this type of deficit is usually not auditory-specific but, rather, focuses on expressive language and planning or organization skills.

These are just a few of the types of auditory training activities that may be implemented. There are as many different ways to approach auditory training as there are children or adults with APD. Some of these techniques are available commercially in a computer-based format; others require direct interaction between the therapist and the child or adult. Some require specialized equipment; others can be accomplished with just a room and a table. Some children or adults may require more than one of these therapeutic approaches; others may not. Again, the most important factor is that the specific objectives of the therapy should be based on the specific nature of the deficit, and the activities should be individualized for the interests and ability levels of the person being treated.

Computer-Based Therapy Programs   A huge upsurge has recently occurred in computer-based therapy programs for language, learning,
and listening difficulties. Computer-based therapy programs have
several advantages, including ease of administration, ability to manipulate signals in ways that are difficult for a clinician to do with his or
her voice or with other available equipment, provision of systematic
procedures, inclusion of graphics to keep the child or adult engaged,
and the ability to present stimuli rapidly and with increasing levels of
challenge based on the person's performance.

Because of these obvious advantages, computer-based therapy programs are becoming extremely popular. However, it is important to
realize that, with communication disorders, an integral part of therapy
must be communication. Therefore, computer-based technology will
never completely do away with the need for therapist-client interaction. It is also important to realize that no one computer-based program will ever be the cure for all types of APD.

Many commercially available computer-based programs have been
used for children and adults with APD, and I have no doubt that
many more will appear in the near future. Many of these programs
have titles that include words such as *listening* or *brain training*. Any or
all of them may be helpful for certain types of APD. At present, however, two programs bear mention because they lead the pack in name
recognition and popularity: Fast ForWord and Earobics. We should
also briefly consider a third popular therapy program that is not
computer-based but operates on similar principles—Auditory Integration Therapy.

- **Fast ForWord®** (FFW; **Scientific Learning Corporation;**
  www.scilearn.com). Originally designed to address language
  learning impairments in children, FFW was based largely on the
  research of Dr. Paula Tallal of Rutgers University and Dr.
  Michael Merzenich of the University of California at San Fran-
  cisco. Because APD has been considered a contributing factor to

many language learning impairments, FFW has become a popular method of treating APD in children. The theory behind FFW is that many of these children have problems processing information that occurs very rapidly and, therefore, require speech to be presented at much slower rates before they can understand the message. The program trains speech-sound processing by systematically altering both the timing and loudness of key acoustic features, and by increasing the complexity of what the listener is able to process. The activities are presented in a series of games that are visually engaging and that provide reinforcement immediately following each response. In short, FFW retrains the brain to hear speech sounds more clearly and rapidly so that the person with language learning impairments can process, and therefore understand, more easily. It also targets other types of receptive language abilities. Candidacy for FFW requires the administration of a specific battery of tests, and the program must be administered by a clinician certified in FFW. Supplemental programs now take the first version of FFW to higher, more complex levels.

I have seen many children with APD, particularly those with Auditory Decoding Deficit, do well with the FFW programs. I have also seen many children who do not show significant improvement following FFW training. Unfortunately, it is not clear at present which children are best suited for FFW. The most commonly cited disadvantages of the FFW programs are that they are costly, require a lot of time, and cannot be altered to suit individual needs. Nevertheless, in my current clinical experience, FFW is the most frequently requested therapy program by parents who have heard about it through the press or through other parents of children who have gone through the program. Parents should be aware that, although FFW has led to improvements in some children with language, auditory, and related concerns, this does not mean that it is appropriate for everyone with APD. Professional guidance from those trained in the treatment of APD, rather than anecdotal evidence gathered from friends or acquaintances, should determine whether to use the FFW programs.

- **Earobics®** (**www.cogcon.com**). Earobics is the brainchild of Cognitive Concepts, Inc. This computer-based program trains many different auditory and related skills, including speech-sound processing, auditory memory and sequencing, rhythm and related temporal patterns, following directions of increasing linguistic complexity, sound-letter association, and phonological awareness. A recent study had nondisordered children in the Chicago public schools use Earobics as part of their daily academic routine. These children demonstrated a significant increase in reading and spelling ability. Earobics has also been found useful for a wide variety of auditory processing deficits, likely because it trains a wide variety of auditory skills. Earobics is available in three levels: young children, older children, and adolescents/adults. It provides engaging age-appropriate graphics and immediate reinforcement. It is also available in both parent and professional formats, for both home and clinic use.

  There are no candidacy or certification requirements for the Earobics program, and program details can be manipulated by the clinician. For example, the program can be altered to require the child to imitate the stimuli verbally, rather than merely clicking the mouse, thus working on perception and production at the same time. I have found Earobics to be most beneficial when it is employed in a time-intensive manner similar to that suggested by FFW; that is, one hour per day, five days a week, for six weeks. However, there is no recommended ideal at present for the length or intensity of Earobics training. Finally, just as with FFW, it is not yet clear which children or adults will benefit most from the program. Therefore, as with any therapy program, we should not assume that Earobics is appropriate for everyone with APD. Finally, it is possible that, as some researchers have hypothesized, the improvement seen in auditory skills as a result of FFW, Earobics, or similar programs has far less to do with the specifics of the programs but rather is due to an "auditory vigilance" effect. In other words, simply engaging in any challenging auditory activity daily for an extended period of time will result in improvement in auditory skills because we are stimulating auditory areas of the brain. This is an intriguing hypothesis, but one that needs to be researched further before any conclusions can be drawn.

- **Auditory Integration Therapy (AIT).** AIT has recently become popular among laypersons because of anecdotal reports that it improves auditory processing skills. Although not a computer-based program, AIT involves the presentation of ten hours of very loud, pitch-altered (or distorted) music through headphones. The loudness of the music is altered randomly. The theory behind AIT is that it remediates hearing "distortions" that impair speech-sound discrimination and recognition by making the inner ear work harder. This theory has met with a great deal of skepticism by the scientific community, as there does not seem to be any anatomical or neurophysiological basis for these assertions. Although some evidence suggests that AIT may be useful for some children with autism, a recent study conducted by Karen Yencer at the State University of New York at Buffalo does not support the benefit of AIT for children with auditory processing deficits. Indeed, there is some possible harm associated with the procedure in that some children who have undergone AIT are unable to listen to music via headphones thereafter. Many of the relevant professional organizations—the American Speech-Language-Hearing Association, American Academy of Audiology, and the Educational Audiology Association—consider AIT experimental. Because of these concerns, along with the lack of a scientific basis and data to support the efficacy of AIT, I do not recommend this program for people with APD, even though it appears to enjoy much popular support from laypersons.

It is important to weigh carefully the potential costs and benefits of any new therapy program. Professional advice should be sought to augment anecdotal claims from parents and other supporters of a program and to help people with APD evaluate scientific claims made by the program's creators. If side effects, such as ringing in the ears, inability to listen to music via earphones, or discomfort, occur during or after any therapy session with a given program—especially one that uses very loud sounds—the possibility of ear damage should be considered. As a general rule, I do not recommend programs that may potentially harm the ear.

Home-Based Therapy Programs In some cases of APD, especially in children, additional therapy may be indicated over and above that which is provided by the school system or the private therapist. Luckily, many intervention techniques, some of them computer-based, can be implemented easily and affordably at home, with appropriate guidance from professionals in determining which techniques would be most appropriate.

Several issues must be considered before beginning any home-based therapy. One of the most important is cost, both in money and time. Some formalized, computer-based therapy programs designed or adapted for use in the home require specialized training, supervision by a certified professional, and expensive software. These programs may also require parents to travel for training. Some of these programs can cost thousands of dollars, and not all programs are covered by private medical insurance. Moreover, many of these programs require up to two hours of daily training, with time inevitably taken away from spouses, other family members, and more enjoyable activities. These costs, money and time, may, indeed, be prohibitive. The relative benefits should be carefully researched and weighed before entering into home-based therapy. Parents should always explore possible alternative, less costly programs that might nevertheless be just as effective.

A second critical consideration should be the nature of the therapy activities implemented in the home. Parents should always have professional guidance on which home-based therapy activities are appropriate for their child. Seeking information and support from other parents of children with APD is invaluable in helping parents understand and cope with a child's auditory deficit. However, other parents of children with APD—no matter how well-informed—are not qualified to recommend specific therapies for your child. It does not matter how effective a particular program may have been for a friend's child. Only a trained professional can determine whether it is appropriate for your own child's unique circumstances and deficit.

Finally, therapy in the home should be made as enjoyable as possible and not approached as a necessary evil that is forced upon the child. Approaches that masquerade as games, especially those that can involve the whole family, are preferable to those that isolate the child from other family members or that appear too similar to the hard work required at school or in the clinic. Here are some activities that can be implemented in a fun, enjoyable manner in the home:

1. For children with Auditory Decoding Deficit, especially those who also have spelling or reading problems, games that involve phonological awareness and sound-symbol association can be used as therapy tools. For example, games such as Scrabble (the regular or Junior version, depending on the spelling level of the child) can be enjoyed by the whole family. A team approach is recommended so that the child with APD is not left alone in his or her efforts, and focus should be taken away from winning and placed on enjoying the playing of the game. For very young children who are struggling with discriminating between speech

sounds (such as *da* versus *ga*), games such as duck-duck-goose can be played in which the words *duck* and *goose* are replaced with the problematic speech sounds (e.g., *da-da-da-da-GA!*).

2. For children with Prosodic Deficit, reading aloud as a family (dramatically exaggerating the characters' utterances to make tone-of-voice cues more apparent) can be both fun and instructive. Family members can take turns reading from a popular book and can even act out various parts. Charades is also useful for training skills related to perception of nonverbal body and facial cues. And it's fun! Simon Says helps children listen for key words in a message. Finally, social communication skills can be worked on by having the whole family engage in role-playing, puppet shows, or mini-plays in which different social situations are acted out.

3. Children with Integration Deficit can benefit from any activity that forces the two hemispheres of the brain to work together. A huge variety of activities fit the bill, almost all of which are fun and can be enjoyed by the whole family. Family members might vote to learn to juggle, play soccer, or learn how to play the piano. Video games that require rapid responses from both hands to visual targets that appear from the sides of the screen (such as many of the space wars shoot-'em-up games) can challenge and improve interhemispheric skills. Remember, however, that these activities are likely to be difficult for the child with Integration Deficit. Therefore, parents should watch closely for signs of frustration. Once again, make sure that the focus is not on winning or being the best player, but on having fun.

4. Scavenger hunts are a great activity for children with Associative Deficit. Instructions and clues can be given that increase in length and complexity as the child becomes better at following directions. Parents should make sure that successful completion

of each step is reward, and that everyone who plays earns the same rewards, not just the child with APD. Family members should take turns rather than all working on the same clue at the same time so that competition is kept to a minimum, particularly since the child with Associative Deficit is likely to be much slower at following each direction. Scavenger hunts are also appropriate for children with Output-Organization Deficit, as are games that challenge memory, sequencing, and action, such as Concentration or the electronic memory and sequencing game Simon.

Obtaining APD Therapy Through the School System

- **Determining when direct therapy services are needed.** For many children with APD, classroom modifications will improve access to the information presented, but will not address the child's difficulties in specific academic and communication skill areas. In addition, we should always keep in mind that today most classrooms have from fifteen to thirty students and only one teacher. Sometimes, the teacher may have an aide, but not always. Within that classroom, several children may have special needs. All of these children deserve an appropriate education. This places an enormous burden on the classroom teacher, who must try to meet the individual needs of every child in the classroom and, at the same time, teach the lesson effectively. This is particularly difficult when children with vastly different needs are placed in the same classroom.

   Therefore, in many situations, direct special education or related services may be indicated. Depending on the particular difficulties a child is having, tutoring in reading, spelling, mathematics, and other subjects might be required. Resource-room special-education teachers may be enlisted for one-on-one or small-group therapy outside the classroom. They may also come

into the classroom itself to assist children. Although some parents worry that their children will miss important information if
they are taken from the classroom for "pull-out" services, this is
often the most effective way of addressing a child's problem
areas. The skills learned in these sessions may then be generalized to the classroom through in-room assistance.

Children with APD may also require related services such as
speech- or language-based therapy by the school speech-language
pathologist. Again, this therapy often consists of a combination
of in-room intervention and individual or small-group pull-out
therapy.

Finally, other special-education-related services, such as occupational or physical therapy or psychological services, might be
indicated for some children with APD, particularly those with
cross-modality or social-emotional-behavioral difficulties.

The services a child receives should be matched to his or her
difficulties. The child with Auditory Decoding Deficit, for example, may receive direct training in phonological awareness skills by
the speech-language pathologist. Or phonological awareness
skills might be incorporated into reading and spelling intervention by the resource-room teacher or tutor. The child with
Prosodic Deficit may receive direct therapy for social communication skills and extracting key words from the ongoing message.
This therapy may be done by the speech-language pathologist or
by a combination of providers working as a team. The team may
include a psychologist to address the child's social and emotional
concerns, whereas resource-room assistance may focus on math
skills or other academic areas.

The child with Integration Deficit often receives occupational
or physical therapy to help with coordinating both hands or both
feet, integrating multimodality information, and similar abilities.
The child with Associative Deficit may receive therapy focusing
on receptive language skills, following directions, and compre-

hension of more complex language forms. The child with Output-Organization Deficit may work on expressive language skills in both speaking and writing and may receive occupational or physical therapy for motor skills, as well.

My experience has been that it is more efficient and effective to approach therapy as a team effort than to piecemeal it into small, seemingly unrelated chunks. For example, aspects of phonological awareness may be incorporated into existing reading and spelling intervention sessions when a child is diagnosed with Auditory Decoding Deficit. In this manner, the speech-sound awareness activities are an integral part of reading and spelling right from the outset, rather than a separate "listening" skill that must then be related to the written word. Expressive language, written language, and handwriting are all somewhat related abilities and can be worked on together by the resource-room teacher, speech-language pathologist, or other appropriate service provider. This approach not only saves time—on the part of the service providers and the child—but also helps the child tie the individual skills together and generalize them to nontherapy situations.

- **Navigating the legal jungle and obtaining school-based special-education services.** The type of any direct special education or related services and the amount of time that will be devoted to these services are determined by the multidisciplinary child study team for each child individually. Parents are integral parts of that team, but so are the classroom teacher, speech-language pathologist, audiologist, psychologist, special education or resource-room teacher, social worker, occupational and physical therapist, and any other appropriate service provider. The need for special education and related services is determined by the team as a whole. For children to obtain these types of services in the schools, they must first be eligible for special education. This determination is made on the basis of guidelines set forth in current federal law, with specific definitions and details determined at the state or local level.

Before this determination is made and services can be obtained, several steps must be completed:

1. Someone (the parent, teacher, or other individual) raises a concern about the child's academic or communicative performance or other difficulties the child seems to be having. Special education services cannot begin until a full evaluation has been completed and the child has been judged eligible. When a concern is raised, this is pretty much the same as asking for an evaluation. Parents should request an evaluation in writing. Often a prereferral meeting will occur, including classroom and special education or resource teachers, speech-language pathologists, audiologists, psychologists, and anyone else who would be appropriate. Based on the nature and severity of the concern, the decision will be made whether to (1) refer the child for special education consideration and assessment (which cannot occur without a parent's permission), (2) implement some classroom and related modifications (which do not require a special education classification), or (3) keep an eye on the child and reconvene later to reconsider the matter, if needed.

2. The types of evaluations that will be conducted will depend on the types of difficulties the child is having. Sometimes, parents may have had the child tested elsewhere, such as at a private clinic. This information is very important to the multidisciplinary team. However, they may wish to do additional testing in some areas through the school district. It is important that everyone cooperate so that a full evaluation can be obtained to determine whether the child qualifies for special

education services. Eligibility must be determined within forty-five days of the initial referral for evaluation.

3. Once a child is judged eligible for special education services, the multidisciplinary team will meet again to develop an individualized education plan (IEP). The IEP must be developed within thirty days of the determination of eligibility. This plan is a contract that sets forth the specific services the child will receive and where (e.g., individualized or small-group therapy, in-classroom assistance), and the amount of time per week that will be spent in related services. Classroom accommodations, special considerations, and all other aspects of the child's educational needs are addressed in the IEP. Specific goals and objectives, along with activities to attain those goals and criteria for measuring progress, are identified. The IEP is reviewed every year, and the child is reevaluated thoroughly every three years (referred to as a *triennial evaluation*) to, once again, determine current functioning levels and special education eligibility. Parental permission and signatures are not required for the triennial evaluation unless the child's disability category or eligibility for services is being changed.

4. For infants and toddlers, the procedure is similar; however, the outcome is an individualized family service plan (IFSP), which is a family-centered management plan. This plan must be developed within forty-five days of referral for special education, be reviewed every six months, and should include a transition plan for children entering preschool.

- **Determining eligibility for special education services.** Our current special education laws have their basis in the landmark civil rights case *Brown vs. Board of Education*, outlawing segregation in public schools, decided by the U.S. Supreme Court in 1954. This case led to the Rehabilitation Act of 1973 (now the Americans with Disabilities Act), which prohibits discrimination against people with disabilities if they are employed by a federal government contractor or the federal government itself, or if they are involved in activities that are federally funded. Schools fall into this latter category.

In 1975, the Education for All Handicapped Children Act was passed. This act has gone through several revisions since 1975 and is currently referred to as the Individuals with Disabilities Education Act (IDEA). IDEA was reauthorized by Congress in 1997 and is the basis for all special education law in the United States.

Before we examine the provisions of IDEA a little more closely, it is important to realize that this act was very nearly not reauthorized in 1997. In fact, the 104th Congress failed to reauthorize the act, and bills were presented that threatened the very nature of special education services in the United States. Only following an enormous grassroots campaign and significant lobbying by concerned professional and parent organizations was IDEA ultimately signed into law by President Clinton on June 4, 1997.

This historical perspective is important because many people take for granted the special education and related services that are provided through our school system. We must recognize that these provisions are reliant on federal support and funding, and that special education and related statutes must be reauthorized every few years. At any point, federal budget cuts may result in a decrease or even an elimination of the special education services that we have come to expect. All of us must be informed as to proposed federal changes in laws that can affect the education of our children.

IDEA defines a child with a disability as one who has been evaluated and shown to have

1. Mental retardation

2. Hearing impairment, including deafness

3. Speech or language impairment

4. Visual impairment including blindness

5. Serious emotional disturbance

6. Orthopedic impairment

7. Autism

8. Traumatic brain injury

9. Other health impairment (including attention deficit and attention-deficit/hyperactivity disorder)

10. Specific learning disability

11. Deaf-blindness

12. On multiple disabilities

    AND who, because of this condition(s)

13. Needs special education and related services. A child who has one of the disabilities listed above and who only needs related services (such as physical therapy), but not special education services to help him or her learn, is NOT a child with a disability under Part B of IDEA.

14. Children aged three through nine years who are experiencing developmental delays in physical, cognitive, communication, social or emotional, or adaptive (daily living skill) development, AND who need special education and related services because of these delays, are also considered disabled under Part B of IDEA.

APD is not included in the IDEA definition of a child with a disability. Furthermore, although the wording of IDEA sets forth general definitions of each of these disabilities, the criteria for whether special education services are needed are set at the state or local level. IDEA states that the disability must "adversely affect educational performance," but no definition is provided for what constitutes an adverse effect. This decision is left up to each individual state. As a result, a child may clearly and reliably have been diagnosed with a disability, as defined by IDEA, but still not qualify for special education services in a given state if he or she does not meet that state's eligibility criteria.

Perhaps an example will make this clearer. A child may do well in math, but be struggling with reading. Depending on the state, specific criteria must be met for the child to be eligible for special education. In some states, it must be demonstrated that a significant discrepancy exists between cognitive capacity and reading achievement, or between academic achievement in other areas and reading achievement. A significant discrepancy may be a certain point spread or percentage difference on standardized tests or other measures, or it may be differences in letter grades, or some other specific criteria. The actual numbers and additional details will differ from state to state. Even if the child has difficulties with reading, he or she will not qualify for special education services unless the specific criteria set forth in that state are met.

Another example is that of a child who has a hearing loss but still exhibits normal language and learning abilities. This is not uncommon for some children who have relatively mild losses or who received hearing aids early in life, allowing them to learn language normally. In this case, the child will not qualify for services under IDEA, even though he or she has a documented physical disability, because *special education* is not required. On the other hand, if the hearing loss adversely affects the child's educational performance (as defined by the state), that same child would be eligible for services.

For the child with APD, state definitions become important. APD alone is not a disability under IDEA. Therefore, APD doesn't appear at all in the eligibility criteria for some states. In others, "auditory processing" or "listening comprehension" is included *under* speech and language impairment, learning disability, or other categories. However, the child with APD must meet the eligibility criteria *for that overriding category* to be considered for special education services. That is, a child with an APD must *also* demonstrate an educationally significant (as defined by the particular state) speech or language impairment, learning disability, or other disability before the child will be eligible for special education.

For parents of children with APD, these rules may seem unnecessarily restrictive and harsh. However, they make more sense when one considers that a limited amount of funding is available for special education and related services in a given state. These funds are distributed among schools and districts based on the number of students who meet the state-defined criteria for special education services. Although the federal government mandates that states provide these services, it provides only limited funds to states for the implementation of IDEA. The states themselves must then figure out how to comply with federal law. As a result, there is a limited amount of money with relatively few qualified service providers to go around. Stated bluntly, funding is incredibly low and caseloads are unbelievably high. Because of these restrictions, provision of special education and related services must be decided very, very carefully, and state rules and criteria must be adhered to.

- **When parents and school districts don't agree.** Once a child is determined to be eligible for special education and related services, the IEP (or IFSP) is drawn up. The details of the IEP should be a team decision. The parents are critical members of the team. Sometimes, however, parents do not agree with the recommendations made by the rest of the team. One of the most common disagreements between parents and service providers is over the amount of direct therapy services that should be provided for the child. In many cases, the parent may feel that daily, one-on-one instruction is indicated, whereas the team feels that two thirty-minute sessions per week are sufficient. The parents may feel that the school doesn't really want to help the child, but is merely going through the motions.

Parents must realize that the provisions of IDEA do not mandate that every child should receive optimum benefit from education. Rather, the provisions state that children with disabilities should be provided sufficient services for them to obtain *reasonable* benefit. In other words, although daily one-on-one instruction or therapy will certainly benefit most children more than will less intense intervention, the school is required only to provide reasonable services. The service providers must consider the needs of all children in their caseloads and divide their time and attention so that each child receives reasonable benefit from special education and related services.

I often describe this critical distinction in the following manner: I could buy a Cadillac for one child or Hondas for several children. There is no doubt that the Cadillac is a better car, but both types of automobile will get the child from one location to another. The Cadillac may be optimum, but the Honda is certainly reasonable. School districts are not required by law to provide a Cadillac for every child, nor can they when they are dealing with limited funds and time. They are, however, required to provide reasonable services—in this example, a Honda—to all children for whom such services are indicated. They are also required to make sure that the child receives reasonable benefit from that Honda. The Honda must be sufficient to assist the child in meeting the goals and objectives set forth in the IEP. Thus, when more intensive services are requested by the parent but denied by the school, it really is not a matter of the school's not wanting to help a child. I rarely encounter a school that does not want to assist a child in the best way possible. When these decisions are made by the IEP team, they usually represent the need to comply with the requirements of federal law while, at the same time, serving all children to the best of their ability with the limited resources they have. Parents may wish their child to receive more intensive services, daily tutoring, or other interventions that are not felt to be necessary by the rest of the team for the child to reach the goals and objectives set forth in the IEP. The responsibility for obtaining and paying for those extra services will probably fall to the parents and not to the school.

It is best for all concerned, especially the child, when the parents and the educational team cooperate and agree. However, sometimes an impasse is reached and the parents reject the IEP. When that happens, the previous IEP remains in effect until an agreed-upon IEP can be developed. If this is the first IEP meeting and no prior IEP was in place, services may be placed on hold or an "interim plan" may be developed.

When parents disagree with the suggestions of the educational team and the team is unwilling or unable to comply with their requests, parents have two primary avenues available. The first is *mediation,* an informal process in which an impartial "judge" is brought in to assist the educational team and the parents reach a solution.

If mediation fails, parents have the right under IDEA to take the school to court in a *due process hearing.* The hearing must be scheduled within thirty-five days of formal, written notification of a parent's intent to pursue such a hearing. After weighing the evidence from both sides at the hearing, an impartial hearing officer makes the final decision.

Due process can be expensive, both in money and emotional impact. For this reason, it is always more desirable for parents and schools to reach mutually acceptable solutions through collaboration or mediation. However, it's important for parents to know that they do have the right to due process if the need arises, but they must pursue it carefully and upon legal advice.

We have barely scratched the surface of the provisions of IDEA and how it affects managing children with disabilities, including APD, in the schools. We have not explored many facets of the legal jungle, such as timelines that must be adhered to, loopholes that should be identified, rights and responsibilities of both the parents and the schools that will impact services to the child. I strongly encourage parents of children with APD to become familiar with the provisions and mandates of IDEA. In my experience, many of the misunderstandings that arise between parents and schools are due to parents' lack of information about what the laws actually say and what their rights and responsibilities are. There are several resources and Web sites for parents regarding interpretation and implementation of IDEA. One that I have found particularly useful is the parent-friendly Web site www.ideapractices.com.

- **What to do when a child does not qualify for special education services.** The Americans with Disabilities Act of 1990 (ADA) prohibits discrimination against anyone with a disability by any employer, not just those receiving federal funds. Section 504 states that schools must make adequate accommodations for students with disabilities so that they have equal access to educational services. Some children with APD who do not qualify for special education services may still need certain accommodations in the classroom. For example, an assistive listening device, preferential seating, note-taker, and other environmental modifications may be considered under a 504 plan. To obtain these accommodations, it must be shown that the student has a disability that limits a daily life function (for example, learning or communication) and that each accommodation is necessary for the child to access education. The 504 plan will delineate the necessary accommodations, and the plan should be reviewed periodically. Direct special education and related services, such as speech-language therapy, are not considered accommodations under a 504 plan.

Parents should realize that a child diagnosed with APD may not qualify for services through their local school district. Even when a child does qualify for school-based services, these services may need to be augmented with private or home-based therapy—a responsibility that rests upon the parents' shoulders.

Direct therapy is a critical part of the overall management plan for a person with APD. However, all too often, it is taken to the extreme. When a child exhibits a disorder such as APD, sometimes all attention and focus is on the child's difficulties and means of remediating them. The result is that, for many children with APD, life becomes one big therapy session. I have worked with children who spend all day at school, often followed by clinic-based therapy sessions, only to go home, eat dinner, complete their homework, and *then* spend another hour and a half in yet more therapy activities. These children are exhausted mentally, emotionally, and physically.

Therapy should be regular, challenging, and intensive. But it must also be realistic. Parents should always be alert to signs of impending breakdown in the child. These may include refusing to participate, crying, exhibiting a lack of progress or even a regression in skills, sullenness, and withdrawal. Don't force the child to work, work, work all the time. And try to avoid cajoling the child with the statement "This is best for you." Parents should always remember that childhood lasts but a few short years, and that the responsibilities of adulthood set in all too soon. Children with APD must be allowed time just to be children, to build memories that are separate from the disorder, and to do things that don't have any real purpose—things that are done just for the sheer joy of it. We must always be aware that an extreme focus on therapy can rob a child of the very act of being a child.

Therapy for APD can be undertaken with people of all ages. The most important factor, however, is to make sure that all environmental modifications and direct treatment recommendations are based on the unique characteristics of the person's disorder and his or her individual life circumstances. But even when environmental modifications and remediation activities are appropriately implemented, people with APD may still have some residual listening difficulties that will persist for the remainder of their lives. The third and final component of APD management is the teaching of compensatory strategies—what I call "living with APD."

7

LIVING WITH APD

APD IS NOT A disease. You can't take a pill to cure it. Although direct therapy may eradicate the disorder in some people, it is difficult to predict how much someone will benefit from treatment. Certainly, the amount of effort put forth is one factor, but other factors may include the age of the person (the younger the better), the type and severity of the deficit, the underlying biological cause of the disorder, and the brain's individual capacity for change. We still do not know why some people with APD can have it successfully remediated (or seem to grow out of the disorder), while others cannot. The fact is, many people with APD will continue to experience some degree of the disorder for the rest of their lives.

It's not all bad news, however. Just as environmental modifications and direct treatment can alleviate some of the symptoms of APD, so can compensatory strategies help the person to live, learn, and communicate successfully. These compensatory strategies, drawn from higher-order cognitive and language skills, will help the person with APD to listen better and to take charge of his own comprehension.

The use of compensatory strategies will also render specific auditory treatment more effective—if those strategies are employed at the same time as auditory training. There is a good reason for this. Our ability to understand spoken language relies on many different skills and levels of processing, all of which operate simultaneously. To understand and communicate effectively, we must be able to hear the message, discriminate among similar-sounding elements, put meaning to the words or sounds, follow the syntax or linguistic structure, and read social communication cues. First and foremost, however, we must be actively engaged in listening. A truly comprehensive management program will address all of these factors and will focus on strengthening those higher-level skills that, while not auditory-specific, can nevertheless affect how well someone listens and understands. Approaching APD management in this comprehensive, holistic manner helps the person with APD get more out of the direct auditory training activities while, at the same time, it teaches methods of improving comprehension in the real world.

I must acknowledge two experts in the field of APD whose research has helped to shape our current management approaches: Dr. Gail Chermak, Chair of the Department of Speech and Hearing Sciences at Washington State University, Pullman; and Dr. Frank Musiek, Director of Audiology at the Dartmouth-Hitchcock Medical Center in Lebanon, New Hampshire. Much of the information in this chapter is based on their years of work managing APD in children and adults.

TAKING THE INITIATIVE: BECOMING AN ACTIVE LISTENER

Anyone who has lived with APD for a long time may eventually become a "passive" listener. Dealing regularly with miscommunications, misunderstandings, and the exhaustion that occurs from putting so much effort into something that is often unsuccessful can lead to withdrawal from social situations, decreased motivation to participate in discussions, and fewer attempts to clarify messages that are not heard or understood correctly. For any listener, the degree of motivation and effort put into hearing, comprehending, and participating in communication has a great deal to do with how successful the listener is. These factors are even more important for people with APD, because they must put forth more effort than the average listener to reap the same rewards. Therefore, learning how to listen actively is a critical skill for any child or adult with APD.

All of us need to put some effort into communicating effectively. All of us have misunderstood a message or missed it entirely because we weren't paying attention, our minds were elsewhere, or we were bored with the conversation. Our own lack of effort and attention led to the miscommunication, and failure cannot be blamed on the speaker or the listening environment.

One of the first steps in becoming an active listener is to take responsibility for our own listening successes or failures. People with APD must be taught to recognize and actively manipulate those factors that are under their control. All too often, they feel helpless and unable to bring about any greater listening success. Over time, they may stop trying altogether, or they may learn to blame every misunderstanding on the disorder, rather than acknowledging that their own lack of motivation and effort may have played a part. They may be unaware, or be unwilling to admit, that they could have done some things themselves to enhance their chances of success.

Research into active listening has shown that the more we involve our entire bodies—not just our ears—in listening, the better we are able to understand what is said. In other words, where the body goes, the ears (and mind) follow. This "whole body listening" approach suggests that, to get the most from a spoken message, the listener should

- Sit (or stand) up straight so that the body is alert rather than slouching in a chair or relaxing against a wall

- Lean the upper body or incline the head slightly toward the speaker in undivided attention

- Keep the eyes firmly fixed on the speaker, watching while listening

- Eliminate unnecessary movement, including foot swinging, finger-tapping, leg bouncing, or any other motion that can divert attention from the speaker

- Avoid any other task while listening, such as watching television, reading a newspaper, or following along in a textbook

- Forcefully bring back attention whenever the mind begins to wander

Recently, I worked with a high school boy with APD. Although he clearly exhibited an auditory deficit that interfered with his ability to understand lectures, his lack of motivation and effort made the situation worse. Kevin earned far better grades in his science class than he did in civics, although both classes were lecture-based. When pressed, Kevin admitted that civics bored him and that he often found himself making plans for the weekend or thinking of something else during class. The benefits of environmental modifications and auditory skills training were then basically wasted because Kevin was not employing any of the techniques he had learned. We worked with Kevin to admit that a large part of his failure in civics was due to his own lack of motivation and effort rather than to the disorder itself. He was taught how to listen with his whole body, and even though civics continued to bore him, his grades improved significantly once he began to take responsibility for his own listening behaviors.

In Kevin's case, he also revealed that he liked to study with music playing in the background. This is not uncommon, and recent studies have shown that music can, indeed, enhance learning and studying. However, Kevin liked to listen to rock music with a great beat and good lyrics. A drummer in his school band, Kevin admitted that he often found himself drumming (and sometimes even singing) along with the music while he was reading his assignments in civics or science or some other class. Although he insisted that this helped him to study, his comprehension of what he had read suggested otherwise.

Remember, where the body goes, the mind follows. Tapping his foot or drumming his hand probably diverted some of Kevin's attention away from what he was reading. Singing to the music certainly diverted his attention. To illustrate this point, I asked Kevin if he liked to listen to music while he drove a car (in our state, the legal driving age is fourteen, and Kevin had been driving for almost three years by this point). Of course, he said yes. And like many of us, he liked his driving music to have a beat. His taste in music was pretty eclectic: a little Springsteen here, a little Eminem there. And like most teenagers, he liked to listen to it loud.

Then, I asked him what was the first thing he did when he hit a construction area or an area of heavier traffic where cars were slowing down ahead of him. After thinking about this for a moment or so, Kevin's eyes opened wide in surprise. "I turn down the radio," he said.

And that is exactly what most of us do when we really need to concentrate. No matter how much we like our music, our first action when we need to concentrate on our driving or are looking for a street address is usually to turn down the volume, even though driving in traffic or looking for an address are visual acts that don't require our hearing at all. Just the act of turning down the volume tells us that we are aware on some subconscious level that the music is interfering with our ability to concentrate.

I suggested that, if Kevin wanted to listen to music while he was studying, he should choose those types of music that have been shown to focus, rather than divert, attention: soft classical, New Age, and other music that is not intrusive and that flows gently in the background. As a general rule, music that makes us want to tap our feet or get up and dance doesn't help concentration. When Kevin agreed to do away with the rock music while he was studying, his ability to understand and remember what he had read improved immediately. He was, in turn, more familiar with the information when it arose during lectures, and his understanding of the lectures improved that much more.

My good friend and colleague Dr. Jeanane Ferre emphasizes the need for whole-body listening as a cardinal rule of APD therapy by posting the following sign on her wall: NO DANCING.

Even when we are trying our best to concentrate on what is being said, all of us invariably allow our attention to wander once in a while. When we realize that we are lost and have missed some of what was said, we usually make an effort to catch up, quickly doing some mental backtracking and inferential thinking. Unfortunately, many people with APD who have become passive listeners do not attempt to pick up the thread of the conversation or message once it has been lost. Often, the entire rest of the lecture or conversation is wasted on them from the first point at which attention wandered. This is another factor in active listening that is directly under the listener's control. People with APD must be taught the importance of actively reengaging attention and active listening as soon as they realize that their minds have drifted so that even more information is not missed. Often, this requires giving themselves a mental shake, forcing their minds back on the topic at hand, and consciously engaging in whole-body listening by sitting up straighter and focusing completely on the teacher or speaker.

Finally, becoming an active listener means becoming aware of any other factors that might be interfering with the ability to get the most from listening. If the person with APD cannot see the speaker or is sitting in an area where there is extraneous noise, she should request a seating change or move to another location where listening conditions are better. Likewise, if a conversational partner continually talks to the person with APD while she's performing another task, when there is noise, or when they are not facing one another, the person with APD should alert the speaker of the need for changes. People with APD should never be afraid to ask for repetition or clarification if a message is misunderstood, or even if they just want to make sure that they got the right information.

Active listening requires us to identify those factors in the environment or in ourselves that are interfering with listening or concentrating, and then to attempt to change them. Sometimes this requires assertiveness training, particularly for those who are shy or reluctant to express their needs. It also requires that people with APD take responsibility when the fault for miscommunication or misunderstanding lies within themselves, rather than blaming everything on the disorder. Many people with APD are astounded to learn just how much of the ability to listen and understand is actually under their control. This leads to a sense of self-empowerment and an improvement in self-image and self-esteem. They do not have to be helpless victims of a disorder. They have power over their own listening behaviors, and when listening to and conversing with others.

OPERATING ON A HIGHER PLANE: METACOGNITIVE AND METALINGUISTIC STRATEGIES

We know that a lot more goes into auditory processing than just being able to hear and discriminate the acoustic signal. Bottom-up processing factors, such as hearing loss, certainly affect our ability to understand. Similarly, top-down factors that relate to thinking, language, and planning also affect how we hear and understand. These top-down or *metacognitive* and *metalinguistic* factors can be used to our advantage to get more from an auditory message.

Metacognitive Strategies In a sense, the principles of active listening fall under the category of metacognitive strategies to compensate for APD. That is, we can actively change our own cognitive or attention behaviors to listen more effectively. Other metacognitive strategies that have been shown to be useful for people with APD include:

- **Self-instruction and reauditorization.** In this strategy, the person with APD is taught to "talk out" the steps of a listening task using a step-by-step procedure:

1. At first, the clinician models the target behavior while talking aloud, using statements and questions such as:

   This is a really difficult-to-understand lecture.

   I should sit up straight, watch the speaker, and listen for important, key words.

   What is the main theme or message of the communication?

   What are the key words?

   What do the key words mean and what information can I draw from them?

   Did I miss any information?

   If so, what have I learned or read previously that gives me knowledge to fill in the missing pieces?

   What conclusions can I draw from this message?

   Are my conclusions logically related to the subject at hand?

   Are my conclusions and actions correct?

2. The person with APD performs the task while the clinician talks aloud, using the same statements and questions. In this way, the clinician guides the person with APD through the key points of the message to draw appropriate, accurate conclusions.

3. The person with APD performs the task while self-instructing aloud.

4. The person with APD performs the task while self-instructing quietly (or whispering).

5. The person with APD performs the task while covertly (i.e., silently) self-instructing.

Through these steps, the person with APD is taught to plan in advance what types of information to listen for, how to go about listening for that information, and how to draw conclusions or inferences from the message. Interestingly, some children with APD do this naturally. Often, if you listen carefully, you might hear a child with APD whispering softly to himself as he repeats key information or coaches himself along. The key here is to teach people with APD to do this silently and automatically when they are in difficult listening situations or when they must attend to and remember a significant amount of information. A related strategy, *reauditorization,* simply means repeating key information aloud or silently. We have all used this strategy when we have looked up a phone number in the telephone book and are trying to remember it en route to the telephone. This strategy can help anyone with APD remember and reinforce multistep directions or other key points of a message.

- **Self-regulation and problem-solving.** In self-regulation, the person with APD is taught to analyze and problem-solve a difficult communicative situation:

  1. The first step in this process is to analyze the situation and identify the nature of the problem. For example, is the student having difficulty hearing the teacher?

  2. An appropriate goal is set for solving the problem. If the student is having difficulty hearing the teacher, then an appropriate goal would be to hear the teacher better.

  3. A plan of action is devised for accomplishing the goal. If a hissing radiator is nearby, perhaps moving to a different location might be an appropriate action for accomplishing the goal of hearing better.

  4. The plan of action is put into effect and the results are evaluated. Did moving away from the radiator and closer to the teacher help the student hear better? If so, then the plan was appropriate and the problem was solved. The student can now give herself a pat on the back! If not, perhaps a different plan of attack is in order.

  Approaching communicative problems in this manner teaches the person with APD to look within for solutions rather than to expect someone else to identify and solve the problem. It leads to active, rather than passive, listening and learning behaviors and generalizes to virtually any situation.

- **Self-reflection and journaling.** Some people with APD, especially those who are just learning effective problem-solving strategies, have difficulty identifying and solving a communicative problem while the communication is taking place. Keeping a diary of difficult listening or communication situations and then reflecting on them later can be helpful. The person might carry a small notebook and jot down a line or two following a misunderstanding or miscommunication. Later, he will reflect on the situation—either with guidance by the clinician or alone—and identify the factors that led to the misunderstanding. Then, a plan of action will be developed (and written down in the diary) to be implemented the next time a similar situation arises. This strategy helps the person with APD plan in advance for difficult communicative situations and have a variety of problem-solving strategies ready for implementation when the need occurs.

Metalinguistic Strategies Just as employing higher-level cognitive and planning skills helps to compensate for auditory difficulties, so does use of higher-order language abilities and experience. These *metalinguistic* strategies help people with APD improve their overall knowledge and use of language concepts to facilitate auditory processing. Some useful metalinguistic strategies include:

- **Listening for key words that suggest relationships between topics or ideas in a message.**

  1. Causal words imply that one idea or topic led to another:
     because
     since
     therefore

2. Words such as *either* and *or* indicate that a choice is to be made, whereas *neither* and *nor* or *and* give the opposite message.

3. Tag words tell the listener what sequence should be followed:
   first
   second
   last
   before
   after

4. The word *if* clearly states that a certain condition must be present before the rest of the message is applicable (e.g., *If* you finish your homework, you may watch television).

5. *However* or *but* suggest that a caveat or warning of an exception is coming.

Paying particular attention to these types of words in a message helps in deciphering its meaning and assists in following directions accurately and sequentially.

- **Using context to fill in missing pieces of the message.** Whether reading or listening, all of us come across words that we either don't hear or don't understand. For example, we might read the sentence "The volcano erupted in a horrible blast of smoke and fire." Even if we are unfamiliar with the word *erupted,* we can draw inferences from the rest of the sentence to help us fill in this missing piece. We might ask ourselves, "What do volcanoes do? Specifically, what do they do that results in smoke and fire?" The answer, of course, is that they blow up. Therefore, the word *erupted* must mean "blow up" or "explode." Teaching people with APD to use their knowledge and vocabularies to achieve auditory closure when they can't hear or are unable to understand parts of the message, rather than just giving up on the message altogether, is very important for maximizing comprehension of spoken messages. In addition, this can help to enhance reading comprehension and to build new vocabulary in children with reading and/or vocabulary deficits associated with APD.

- **Reading cues and drawing inferences.** Many social or communicative situations are familiar enough that we can expect certain things to be said. For example, if we are entering a restaurant and the maître d' approaches us at the door with a smile, we can guess that he will say something like "How many? Smoking or nonsmoking?" Similarly, the man who checks his watch, frowns and shakes his head, puts his wrist near his ear and listens intently, and then approaches us is likely to say something along the lines of "My watch has stopped. Have you got the time?" For people with APD, making predictions or inferences based on nonverbal or body cues and social expectations can be helpful when messages are not heard or understood clearly. Similarly, reading body and facial cues can help people with APD determine the intent of a message, even if they have difficulty interpreting the person's tone of voice. For example, if the speaker is smiling broadly, he is probably not angry, even if we perceive anger in his tone of voice.

- **Rephrasing information.** Just as having the teacher or speaker rephrase information can help people with APD understand a message, teaching the person with APD to say the information in her own words can also help. This strategy will also immediately alert the speaker when a message has been misunderstood. For example, when given a complicated instruction by her supervisor, the person with APD might say, "Let me see if I have this right. You want me to alert the billing department before I type up all of the sales contracts. Correct?" This provides the supervisor with an opportunity either to agree (e.g., "Yes, that's correct") or to avert a potentially disastrous situation (e.g., "No. I want you to type up the contracts first, *then* alert the billing department"). It also allows the person with APD to make sure that she is following the instructions correctly.

This type of strategy works well for school-aged children, too. For example, the child might ask, "So, we are to do all of the odd problems on page twenty-one and the even problems on page twenty-two?" If the teacher responds, "No, you can choose *either* the odd problems on twenty-one *or* the even problems on twenty-two," the child has clarified the instructions and saved both time and effort. Because people with APD are not always aware that they have misunderstood messages, teaching them to rephrase information can be a valuable tool to avoid miscommunications, errors, and wasted time and effort. Moreover, just having the person repeat the message in her own language helps in remembering the information.

PUT IT IN WRITING: MEMORY ENHANCEMENT TECHNIQUES

Who among us wouldn't appreciate tips that might improve our memory? People with APD may be spending so much of their time and energy just understanding a message that remembering it all can be just too much to ask for. But there are tricks to help ensure that what is finally heard and comprehended can actually be retained.

- **Chunking.** Ask another person to listen to you as you read aloud the following series of letters, allowing a two-to-three-second pause between each letter: F...B...I...I...R...S...N... F...L...C...I...A...P...T...A...C...B...S. Now ask the person to recall or repeat as many letters as possible. Chances are, they will only be able to repeat between five and nine of them. This is because our *short-term memory*, or ability to recall information recently presented, only holds about seven (plus or minus two) pieces of information at a time. However, if you know how to *chunk* information together, you could easily repeat the whole list. All it takes is organizing the letters into groups, or chunks, that make logical sense: FBI, IRS, NFL, CIA, PTA, CBS. Now you have only six pieces of information to remember instead of eighteen, and six is within the limits of most people's short-term memory. Teaching people with APD to chunk information is a useful memory tool. For example, when going to the grocery store, they may put similar items into one category. Therefore, instead of trying to remember to buy eggs, cereal, bread, cheese, milk, bagels, hamburger buns, and yogurt, they may group these items into two general categories: dairy (eggs, cheese, milk, and yogurt) and grains (bread, cereal, bagels, and buns).

- **Elaboration.** Another useful memory tool is to assign a meaningful sentence, analogy, or other type of trigger to items that need to be remembered. For example, my son was recently trying to memorize the capitals of each state in the country. The teacher had provided silly little stories to aid in remembering. To remember the capital of Florida, the children just had to think of a man in Florida at a beach: this man goes swimming, and he grabs a towel to dry off when he comes out of the water. Therefore, a towel has he (Tallahassee). Silly, perhaps, but it works. I myself will never forget the definition of *emesis,* which means "vomiting," because my professor in one of my first medical-based undergraduate courses showed a slide of a man yelling at a woman, "Hey, Mrs. [emesis], you just vomited on my floor!"

  Other similar tricks include assigning acronyms, or series of letters, to items needing remembering. A classic example used in neuroanatomy classes everywhere is the sentence "On Old Olympus's Towering Top, A Finn And German Viewed Some Hops" to remember the names of the twelve cranial nerves in the central nervous system. The first letter of each word in the sentence corresponds to the first letter of the name of a nerve. Without this memory device, I doubt any of us would ever have learned the names of the cranial nerves, and I use this sentence even today to help my own recall. Similarly, the name ROY G. BIV has helped schoolchildren everywhere remember the order of the colors of the rainbow: Red, Orange, Yellow, Green, Blue, Indigo, and Violet.

- **Setting it to music.** Some children and adults retain information better if music and/or movement is incorporated into memorization. Probably the most familiar example of this is the "Alphabet Song." Most children learn to sing the ABC's long before they even know what the song means, and this helps them to learn and remember the order of the letters of the alphabet later. Rhymes and songs such as "Pat-a-Cake" and "Itsy Bitsy Spider" are learned easiest when accompanied by the hand motions. Creating rhythms, rhymes, tunes, or hand motions to which new information can be set can help in the initial learning and retention of information, and it is a fun activity for children. However, children with interhemispheric integration deficits may not benefit from this strategy because it employs so many different types of skills all at once.

- **Recoding the information.** One of the best memory strategies is to draw a picture. Although writing down information can also be helpful, drawing a picture does not require the same type of verbal and spelling skills as writing (which may be difficult for people with APD) and also recruits additional areas of the brain that are not necessarily used for linguistic information. Furthermore, drawing a picture requires the listener to summarize the main idea of the message into a single representation, which aids in comprehension. One theory of short-term memory is that we have two primary methods of retaining information for a short time. One of these, the phonological loop, is auditory-dependent and can be activated by verbally rehearsing or repeating the information to oneself. The other, the visual-spatial sketchpad, is the equivalent of drawing a picture in the mind and may be an easier means of remembering for someone with APD. Actually drawing a picture on paper to represent the main idea of a message can help activate the visual-spatial sketchpad. Ultimately, the paper will no longer be needed to recode the information into a pictorial or visual representation in the mind.

WHAT I WANT TO BE WHEN I GROW UP: MAKING REALISTIC LIFE CHOICES

I will never be an Olympic track champion. No matter how hard I practice, I will simply never be able to run fast enough to even come close to making the team. I accept that. I do not consider it a limitation.

Everyone has strengths and weaknesses that help to define them and make them who they are. Our abilities, and our limitations, determine what we can—or cannot—reasonably do. Although we should never limit anyone's dreams unnecessarily or encourage underachievement, people with APD must recognize their limitations and make realistic life choices. It is important for them—indeed, for all of us—to set reasonable goals that can be achieved with hard work and determination.

In my research, I have found that musicians, particularly those who play instruments, such as the piano, that require the coordination of both hands at the same time, demonstrate the best interhemispheric processing abilities. Although this finding seems to suggest that playing a musical instrument can improve our interhemispheric processing skills, another interpretation is equally likely: that people choose to play musical instruments because their interhemispheric processing abilities are good to begin with. In other words, they chose an activity that used their strengths. This *self-selection* process is something that we all do. We gravitate toward those activities at which we feel we can be successful, and away from those that make us feel clumsy or incompetent. To do this, we must identify our own areas of strength and weakness—even if only subconsciously.

Sometimes, parents of children with disabilities, and the people with disabilities themselves, set unrealistically lofty goals. Because so much attention and effort is spent on overcoming their disorder, they may set out not just to succeed at something, but to be the best. Instead of using their personal past performance as a standard for comparison, they are determined to perform better than everyone else. They may sometimes set goals that are far higher than they would be if there were no disorder. As a result, children with APD may be pushed harder than their nondisordered peers, or adults with APD may expect more of themselves than they do of their nondisordered colleagues.

A part of this tendency arises from the need to find internal motivation, to accumulate enough sheer determination to carry through to accomplishments that might otherwise not be achieved. This is a laudable goal. It *is* important for people with a disorder to have a good deal of determination and willingness to work because they may very well need to expend extra effort and time to achieve what others accomplish far more easily. Unfortunately, if taken too far, this mind-set can easily turn out to be a recipe for failure.

Recently, I worked with a little girl whose APD was accompanied by significant learning difficulties in reading, spelling, writing, and other areas. Once her APD had been identified, Ellie threw herself into her therapy sessions with more effort than I had ever seen from a ten-year-old child. And Ellie's effort was not just confined to APD therapy. She also played soccer and softball, took both ballet and karate lessons, and was in the Girl Scouts. Ellie undertook every activity with an air of determination I found somewhat disconcerting in a child her age.

One day, Ellie's mother, bursting with pride, said to me, "Ellie got one hundred percent on her spelling test this week."

Ellie nodded her head, a big smile on her face.

"I am so proud of you!" I exclaimed, hugging her.

Her mother said, "A year ago, she could barely spell her name. Now this! This just goes to show there's nothing she can't do!"

I smiled, but I felt a niggling of concern at the fervent, almost fanatical expression that had begun to appear on Ellie's mother's face.

"This is just the beginning," she went on. "Just watch. Ellie is going to be valedictorian of her senior class. Just wait and see. Isn't that right, honey?"

Ellie nodded in agreement.

"And she'll be a prima ballerina in New York City, won't you, baby?"

Again, Ellie nodded, her determined expression almost matching her mother's. All I could do was watch.

"Nothing's going to stand in the way of my baby. She'll get through this APD thing, and she'll show everyone that no one can tell her what she can or can't do! She'll go to Harvard, be a doctor, win the Nobel Prize. You name it, my daughter will do it!" The mother's voice carried the conviction of a revivalist preacher as she raised her fist in the air. Then, she let out her breath in a deep sigh and hugged her daughter.

I forced an air of nonchalance and simply said. "Well, first things first. Ellie, are you ready for today's session?"

Ellie nodded eagerly, the gleam of determination still shining brightly in her eyes as we walked back to the therapy room.

Of course, it was wonderful to work with a child who was so cooperative and tried so hard during therapy sessions. And I could understand Ellie's mother's need to believe in her child, to motivate her child to work hard and succeed. But in her sincere attempt to cheer her daughter on, I couldn't help but feel that Ellie's mother had made a grave error by grossly overcompensating for her daughter's disorder. Along with applauding Ellie's everyday successes, she had set goals for her daughter that no one, with or without a disorder, could truly be expected to achieve.

There is only one valedictorian. Few girls realize a dream of becoming a prima ballerina. Going to Harvard, becoming a doctor, and winning the Nobel Prize are things that very few people will ever achieve. And Ellie had just been saddled with all three of these goals.

Whether Ellie's mother really expects these things from Ellie is irrelevant. The fact is, Ellie has come to expect these accomplishments from herself, and in her need to please her mother, she may truly believe that she has to achieve these goals to consider herself a success. Each time I speak with Ellie and her mother, these types of comments are reiterated. Certainly, Ellie has come a long way in her therapy and in overcoming her associated learning disabilities. She earns solid grades now—mostly B's, but a few A's here and there—which I feel is an outstanding achievement considering where she began just a few short years ago. She deserves applause, rewards, even brass marching bands for working so hard and coming so far in so short a time.

But Ellie is not satisfied with the progress she has made to date. She is pushing herself toward those other goals, and sometimes I see a vague shadow of frustration—or perhaps fear—on her face when she has difficulty with a task. There is a hint of desperation in the way she throws herself into every activity, attacking it as if it were an enemy. On the one hand, her determination has been a huge factor in her success. But on the other hand, I worry about how she will react when she comes up against a barrier that is insurmountable—as we all do at some point in our lives.

I think that Ellie will be successful by anyone else's standards, and that she will ultimately in large part overcome the disorder that had brought her to me in the first place. But I am not so sure that Ellie will ever be truly satisfied, or truly happy, because the goals that have been set for her—which she has adopted for herself—are so high as to be unreachable for virtually anyone.

Ellie's case may seem extreme but, unfortunately, it is not uncommon. In my practice, I see many parents who are so determined to advocate for their children that they proclaim loudly to the world that their children will not only overcome their disorders but will be the best in anything and everything they do. The need to be the best is a horribly weighty burden for any child to shoulder. For a child with a disorder such as APD, who may be struggling mightily just to run in the middle of the pack, it may prove to be a burden entirely too heavy to bear.

In our society, *average* has become a dirty word. When we are told that we have average abilities or have performed in the average range, we feel disappointed somehow, even though, technically, *average* means that we are right there in the middle of the group—actually, not a bad place to be at all.

For a child or adult with APD who may have been performing in the "well below average" or "deficient" range in many areas, the word *average* is one of the most beautiful words there is. Although our society may have placed unfortunate and undesirable connotations on the word, the child or adult with APD should be allowed to feel pride in this remarkable accomplishment. When someone who has prayed for many years to be "just like all the others" finally overcomes a disorder enough to actually *be* just like all the others, that is something worth applauding. For a child with a significant APD and spelling disorder, earning 100 percent on a spelling test is tantamount to a walk on the moon for a rocket scientist.

In the quest for motivation and determination, in the battle to the death with the beast we call APD, it is critical that everyday accomplishments and efforts be rewarded. It is critical that children's (or adults') performance today be compared to their own performance yesterday or last week or last year, and not to the performance of others. And it is absolutely critical that they know that we will love them, respect them, and support them no matter what. They do not need to be the best, they only need to do *their* best, whatever that may be.

Just as we should set realistic life goals for children with APD, deciding on a career or a work setting requires the same realism. Remember Larry, the man with mild APD who wanted to work on the stock market floor? He couldn't have made a worse choice given his disorder, even though he could have been entirely successful in virtually any other setting. Even I had to take a good, hard look at my strengths and weaknesses and leave a job I loved. In the end, however, I found myself in a job that I loved even more.

When young air force officers want to become pilots, they are required to take a qualifying examination. This exam does not rely on any previous training whatsoever. Instead, it tests to see whether the person has some inherent, automatic processing abilities that can be built upon during pilot training. For example, by looking at drawn representations of the horizon, the person must rapidly decide if an airplane is ascending or descending, banking right or left, based on the angle of the view. I took this test during a brief stint in ROTC in college. I had never had any experience with flying, but I passed. I found it very easy to make these snap judgments. Many of my friends who also took the exam felt the same way. Others, however, left the exam saying, "How on earth could they expect us to know which way the plane is going? We've never done that before!" In other words, they did not have those basic processing abilities that allowed them to perceive those angles automatically, without being taught. What was so effortless for some was extremely difficult for others. In the end, those who failed the test were required to choose another field within the military. Although I passed the examination, I decided not to train as a pilot for other reasons: I don't like heights, and I don't particularly like to fly. I left ROTC and pursued my audiology degree.

Many of us have interests or hobbies that do not necessarily apply to our jobs or careers. What we enjoy in our time off from work might be far less enjoyable if we were forced to do it quickly or daily. Yet, it is important that we find careers or jobs that we can do and that we like. For someone with APD, or any disorder, examining the demands of a job or career before making such a monumental decision is critical. By matching the career choice to his strengths and weaknesses, he can be confident that the job will get done, that success is attainable, and that job satisfaction is possible. Otherwise, he may find himself struggling daily just to perform—which will lead only to frustration and a decrease in self-image and self-esteem.

I will never be an Olympic track champion, but I'm all right with that. I have set my sights elsewhere, toward areas that use my inherent strengths. But that doesn't mean that I can't run like the wind when I want to.

IT TAKES A VILLAGE: RESOURCES FOR CHILDREN AND ADULTS WITH APD

A few years ago, in a small, remote state, several parents and professionals joined together to form a group dedicated to gaining knowledge, funding, and resources for the assessment and management of APD. They brought professionals like myself out to testify in front of state legislators and board of education members about the impact of APD and the importance of accurate diagnosis and treatment. What that relatively small group was able to accomplish was truly amazing. They gained statewide recognition and acknowledgment of the disorder and increased funding in the educational and private systems so that trained professionals could be brought in to consult. Their efforts fostered a degree of interdisciplinary cooperation that I have rarely seen anywhere else before or since.

This experience shows just what can be done when people are willing to work together to fight a disorder such as APD. I have found that much of the resistance to the concept of APD from professionals and others results from lack of education. Adding to this is the misinformation and generalities about APD that are so prevalent right now in the general population. When people learn more about the disorder, when they understand what it is (and what it is not), and when they realize that there are methods of both diagnosing and treating it, they are far more likely to band together for a common cause.

Working together is important not only for the professionals who diagnose or treat APD, but also for parents of children with APD or those with APD themselves. Even the most active of listeners and independent of spirits needs someone to lean on now and then. The need for accurate and appropriate education and support for all of these people is critical. Involving family members and others in APD management is important, but those affected by the disorder need consolation, support, and ideas from others who are living through similar experiences.

At present, few support groups are available for people with APD and their families. For the most part, those that do exist are the result of the efforts of small groups of people in a given locale. Many of these small, local support groups consist of concerned parents who are trying to educate themselves and others about APD, and an unfortunate number of them do not have knowledgeable professionals in their area to consult with. As a result, many myths, inaccuracies, and generalizations about APD have been propagated through these channels, which can often do more harm than good.

The need for a place to turn to for support is great for those affected by APD. The simple comfort of talking to another person who has gone through similar experiences cannot be replaced by any number of professionals or clinicians. The creation of local or regional support groups for APD is a welcome relief for those who are struggling alone.

In response to the need for a national support network for people affected by APD similar to those addressing AD/HD, learning disabilities, and similar disorders, a national clearinghouse for APD information and support has recently been developed. This network is the result of the ongoing efforts of a Florida parent of a child with APD and various professionals and parents throughout the country. The National Coalition for Auditory Processing Disorders, Inc.

(NCAPD) provides information about APD, underwrites on-line support and chat groups, and maintains a database of professionals throughout the country who work with APD. It also provides Web-based simulations of APD and other insightful information.

Along with the NCAPD, our national professional organizations— the American Speech-Language-Hearing Association (ASHA) and the American Academy of Audiology (AAA)—provide accurate, timely information about APD and are useful resources for finding a professional in a given locale.

Still, there is a pressing need for both support and accurate information about this disorder for the general public. The recent upsurge of Web sites and chat groups devoted to APD, along with mention of APD in popular books dealing with learning disorders or related topics, has helped to raise awareness of the disorder. Unfortunately, this increase in awareness is a double-edged sword; much of the information that is currently available through these venues is incomplete or outright inaccurate. In their sincere zeal to help others, people with no particular expertise in APD, other than what they have been told or have experienced, may prescribe treatments for others or suggest diagnostic or therapy approaches that have no basis in science or do not reflect our current knowledge. For this reason, it is critical that support groups throughout the country involve people affected with APD as well as professionals trained in APD diagnosis and management so that these inaccurate perceptions can be corrected and guidance can be provided that is appropriate and reflects current standards.

Auditory processing disorders can affect people of any age, race, socioeconomic status, or gender. They can interfere with language, learning, and communication and can have a devastating impact on the quality of life. Management and treatment of APD require accurate diagnosis of the disorder and a comprehensive understanding of the scientific bases underlying APD as well as the many ways the disorder can affect lives. Although the audiologist is the professional who diagnoses APD, determining how a given APD affects a person's life and planning methods of managing it requires a team approach that involves audiologists, speech-language pathologists, physicians, psychologists, teachers, employers, social workers, parents, family members, and everyone else who is involved with the person at school, at work, or at home.

Following is a short list of resources for people to turn to in their quest to unravel the mystery of APD. Hopefully, this list will grow in the near future as more and more information becomes available on this puzzling, frustrating disorder. Until that time, however, it is important for all of us to work together to spread the word about the many-headed beast we call APD and to encourage professionals and others from all fields to join together in the fight against it. Only then will the misunderstandings, misinformation, misdiagnoses, and cases of mismanagement finally be laid to rest.

American Speech-Language-Hearing Association (ASHA)
10801 Rockville Pike
Rockville, MD 20852
(800) 638–8255
www.asha.org

American Academy of Audiology (AAA)
8300 Greensboro Drive, Suite 750
McLean, VA 22102
(800) AAA-2336
www.audiology.org

National Coalition for Auditory Processing Disorders, Inc. (NCAPD)
P.O. Box 11810
Jacksonville, FL 32239
www.ncapd.org

THE FUTURE
OF APD

OUR KNOWLEDGE OF APD and its causes and effects has grown so rapidly over the past few years that it is almost impossible to predict where the field will be in the next decade. But one thing is certain: no longer will the lack of available information hinder our fight against this many-headed beast. With the latest research focusing on treatments for specific types of APD, earlier and better means of diagnosing APD, and underlying causes of APD, this disorder may no longer be quite so much of a mystery in the near future.

New imaging techniques that allow us to look right into the brain and see how and where functions occur—such as positron-emission tomography (PET) and functional magnetic resonance imaging (fMRI)—are already illuminating things we never knew and confirming things we always suspected about how the brain works. We now know that just the deceptively simple act of listening involves many brain regions, even those that control speech output. As more is learned, it will become increasingly difficult to support a unitary view of auditory processing deficits. Instead, we will be forced to accept that APD can involve many different brain regions and can coexist with disorders in other sensory processing systems.

We may find ourselves once again needing to relabel the disorder. Perhaps we will take the more global view that, in many cases, APD is just the auditory manifestation of a larger central processing disorder that affects other things in addition to listening. As such, even if audiologists remain the professionals qualified to diagnose this auditory piece of the puzzle, we will be forced to include professionals from other disciplines in our endeavors, thus ensuring a multidisciplinary approach to diagnosis and treatment.

I envision a future in which experts in APD come from many different fields and they all undergo the extra training necessary to understand APD in all of its manifestations. No one discipline teaches its students all of the principles necessary for understanding APD. APD crosses discipline boundaries, involving principles of audiology, speech, language, psychology, cognitive neuroscience, learning, and many other areas. Therefore, it requires cross-disciplinary education. Perhaps in the future our APD experts will come from many different walks of life but will have two things in common: accurate knowledge and the sincere desire to do away with artificial disciplinary boundaries and to face the beast head-on in all of its terrible glory.

As more treatment-efficacy research is done, we will be able to predict better who will benefit from specific therapy approaches. The frequency and intensity of therapy that is needed to change listening by reorganizing the brain will be better understood. We will no longer be groping in the dark, searching for even the dimmest ray of hope.

I believe that, if we continue to look for a simple answer to APD, it will continue to elude us. As long as we try to agree on easy, concise definitions, methods of diagnosis, and methods of treatment for APD, we will never reach consensus on anything. The brain is infinitely complex. Any disorder that involves the brain will, likewise, be infinitely complex. Therefore, until we let go of the hope for a simple answer, we may find ourselves never asking the right questions.

We will be able to identify and treat APD better in the near future. We may even agree on what it is and what to call it. But APD will not disappear. It will always occur in children and adults. Every new bit of knowledge, no matter how small, will help us to ensure that future generations do not suffer the misdiagnoses and mismanagement that have characterized our dealings with this disorder in the past.

GLOSSARY

American Academy of Audiology (AAA). The professional organization specifically for audiologists, established in 1988, which provides continuing education opportunities, nonmandatory board certification in audiology, consumer information, and a variety of other functions and services.

American Speech-Language-Hearing Association (ASHA). The professional organization for both speech-language pathologists and audiologists, established in 1925, which oversees accreditation of training programs and the Certification of Clinical Competence (CCC) in both professions and provides continuing education opportunities, consumer information, legislative lobbying, and a variety of other functions and services.

Americans with Disabilities Act (ADA). Based on the Rehabilitation Act of 1973 and enacted in 1990, the ADA protects people with disabilities from discrimination in employment, public services and transportation, public accommodations and commercial facilities, telecommunications, and other areas.

Apgar scores. A tool for evaluating a newborn infant's overall condition after birth. A rating of 0–2 is assigned for each of the following: heart rate, respiratory effort, reflex irritability, muscle tone, and color—with a total possible score of 10. The Apgar is performed at one minute and five minutes after birth, with the second score expected to be higher than the first.

aphasia. A disorder of expressive (speaking) or receptive (understanding) language that arises from damage to specific areas of the brain; a common occurrence following stroke or head trauma.

assistive listening device. Any device designed to help the user hear in difficult or noisy environments; may be used alone or be attached to hearing aids.

Associative Deficit. One of the Bellis/Ferre subtypes of APD; affects the ability to attach meaning and rules to incoming messages, presumably due to dysfunction in or near the auditory association cortex of the brain.

attention-deficit/hyperactivity disorder (AD/HD). A higher-order cognitive or executive-control disorder that involves distractibility and an inability to allocate attention appropriately. Can occur in three forms: predominately inattentive (i.e., without hyperactivity), predominately hyperactive/impulsive, or combined.

audiogram. A graphic representation of a person's hearing thresholds, or the softest sounds he responds to, for various frequencies (or pitches).

audiologist. A specialist in hearing and its disorders. Audiologists are currently required to hold at least a master's degree in audiology for clinical certification through ASHA and board certification through AAA; by 2013, a doctorate (either a Ph.D. or the doctor of audiology, Au.D.) will be necessary for entry into clinical practice.

audiology. The scientific and clinical study of hearing and its disorders.

auditory association cortex. The area in the temporal lobe in which meaning is attached to words or sounds; involves the integration of input from other brain and subcortical areas.

auditory brainstem response (ABR). A measure of the electrical activity arising from the auditory nerve and brain stem in response to sound; frequently used as a "hearing" assessment tool or to diagnose disorders affecting the auditory nerve or brain stem. Electrodes are attached to the listener's scalp and the brainstem responses are recorded on a computer screen for analysis.

auditory closure. The ability to fill in the missing pieces when parts of a message are not heard or understood by relying on higher-level language and reasoning skills and contextual cues.

Auditory Decoding Deficit. One of the Bellis/Ferre subtypes of APD; affects the ability to hear and discriminate among speech sounds and to achieve auditory closure; presumably arises from dysfunction in the primary auditory cortex.

auditory discrimination. The ability to tell when two sounds are different.

auditory electrophysiology. General term referring to any of a number of tests involving the recording of electrical activity from the central auditory pathways in response to sound. Electrodes are attached to the listener's scalp and responses are recorded on a computer screen for analysis.

Auditory Integration Therapy (AIT). An auditory training approach purported to treat hypersensitivity in children with learning disabilities, autism, and related disorders; controversial, with limited data supporting its efficacy for children with APD.

auditory neuropathy. A disorder of neural synchrony (or the ability of auditory nerve fibers to fire together in response to sound) that results in hearing loss and significant difficulties understanding speech, especially in noisy environments. Typically diagnosed through the finding of normal otoacoustic emissions (responses from the inner ear) and abnormal auditory brainstem responses, along with other key diagnostic indicators.

autism. A disorder under the diagnostic umbrella of pervasive developmental delay that is characterized by severely impaired ability to interact socially and to communicate with others and the presence of stereotyped, repetitive behaviors.

backing. An articulation error in which a sound is produced near the back of the mouth instead of at the front (e.g., substituting *g* for *d*).

Bellis/Ferre model of APD. A theoretical model proposed by Dr. Teri James Bellis and Dr. Jeanane Ferre in which five subtypes of APD are delineated, each of which arises from dysfunction in different brain regions and leads to different learning, language, and auditory symptoms and complaints. Subtypes include Auditory Decoding Deficit, Prosodic Deficit, Integration Deficit, Associative Deficit, and Output-Organization Deficit.

binaural. Pertaining to both ears, as in binaural hearing aids.

bottom-up processing. Term used in information processing theory to refer to sensory (or "input") processing of the signal from lower to higher levels in the nervous system.

brain stem. Portion of the neural pathways residing at the base of the brain; the brain-stem auditory pathways are those auditory nervous system structures located between the auditory nerve and the thalamus.

Buffalo model of APD. A theoretical model proposed by Dr. Jack Katz in which four subtypes of APD are delineated, each of which results in different learning, language, cognitive, and auditory symptoms and complaints. Subtypes include Decoding, Tolerance-Fading Memory, Integration, and Organization.

central auditory nervous system (CANS). The nerve pathways from the ear into the brain that are responsible for processing auditory input; includes structures in the auditory nerve, brain stem, thalamus, and cortex; central auditory pathways.

central presbycusis. Age-related deterioration in the ability to hear or understand speech as a result of degeneration in the central auditory pathways.

child find. General term referring to the process of identifying children (especially birth to three years of age) with disabilities.

chunking. A memory aid in which items are organized into logical categories to reduce the number of pieces of information to be memorized.

circumlocution. Describing an item or its purpose or providing other information instead of the object's label; often used as a communication strategy when a person has word-finding problems.

comorbidity. Term referred to the situation in which two or more diseases or disorders occur together in the same person.

computerized tomography (CT). Diagnostic X-ray procedure in which a computer measures densities in the brain, then draws a three-dimensional map or representation.

conditioned play audiometry. A method of testing the hearing of children between the ages of approximately three and five years in which the child is taught to make an overt response (such as dropping a block into a box) when a sound is heard.

conduct disorder. A psychiatric condition in which the child persistently violates the rights of others or fails to comply with expected societal norms; may include aggressive conduct that harms other people, nonaggressive conduct that results in property loss or damage, lying or stealing, and serious violations of rules.

corpus callosum. The central nervous system structure that connects the two hemispheres of the brain; consists of a large bundle of nerve fibers.

cortical. Pertaining to the cortex of the brain.

dichotic. The presentation of a different signal to each ear simultaneously.

dyslexia. General term referring to a disorder of reading.

Earobics. A computer-based auditory training program designed by Cognitive Concepts, Inc. for use with people with auditory processing, reading, and related difficulties. Versions are available for young children (aged four to seven years), older children, and adolescents/adults.

Eustachian tube. The tube that connects the middle ear with the back of the throat and equalizes air pressure between the external environment and the middle ear; eustachian tube dysfunction leads to ear infections in many cases.

executive function. General cognitive control processes that relate to the coordination of knowledge with behavior, involving allocation of attention, problem-solving, planning, and decision-making; ensures that the person's behavior is adaptable to the changing demands of the environment.

expansion. Adding to and enriching a child's utterance to enhance his or her exposure to additional, related vocabulary, language, or concepts.

expressive language. General term referring to the formulation and production of spoken, written, manual, or other forms of language.

Fast ForWord (FFW). Computer-based auditory training program designed by Scientific Learning Corporation for use with children with specific language impairments and related disorders; requires administration by a certified provider.

FM system. An assistive listening device that sends sound from a microphone directly to the listener through frequency-modulated (similar to FM radio) waves carried through the air; particularly useful in helping listeners hear in noisy environments.

fronting. An articulation error in which a sound is produced near the front of the mouth instead of at the back (e.g., substituting d for g).

Full Scale IQ. A number score representing overall cognitive ability in both verbal and nonverbal areas derived from subtest scores of the Weschler Intelligence Scale for Children, third edition (WISC-III).

functional magnetic resonance imaging (fMRI). A brain-imaging technique used to measure brain activity during rest or while performing a specific task; involves measuring changes in elements (e.g., iron, oxygen) in the brain during task performance.

gestalt. A structure, configuration, or pattern that is so integrated into one functional unit that the whole cannot be derived simply from the sum of the parts.

Individualized Education Plan (IEP). An annual, individually developed contract for the provision of special education and related services for children with disabilities that adversely affect education; mandated by federal law (IDEA).

Individualized Family Services Plan (IFSP). An individually developed contract for the provision of special education and related services for infants and toddlers with disabilities that emphasizes family involvement; mandated by federal law and updated every six months.

Individuals with Disabilities Education Act (IDEA). Federal law reauthorized by Congress in 1997 that mandates a free and appropriate public education for all children with disabilities that affect their ability to learn; incorporates previous U.S. Public Laws 94-142 and 99-457 and amendments.

Integration Deficit. One of the Bellis/Ferre subtypes of APD; involves a disruption of the ability of the two hemispheres of the brain to work together; presumably arises from dysfunction in the corpus callosum.

interhemispheric integration. The ability of the two hemispheres of the brain to work together.

invented spelling. A popular, phonics-based educational tool for beginning spellers in which words are spelled as they sound.

Joint Committee on Infant Hearing (JCIH). A group composed of audiologists, speech-language pathologists, otolaryngologists, and other professionals that makes recommendations regarding identification of and intervention for hearing loss in infants and other topics related to infant hearing.

Least Restrictive Environment (LRE). Term referring to the placement of children with disabilities, to the maximum extent possible, in environments with peers without disabilities, with placement in self-contained classrooms or schools only when necessary.

localization. The ability to identify the direction from which a stimulus is coming (e.g., sound localization).

magnetic resonance imaging (MRI). A diagnostic imaging procedure in which the patient is placed in a magnetic field and a computer draws a picture of the structure being imaged; useful for looking at the anatomy of the brain and other soft (nonbone) tissue.

mental retardation. Significantly subaverage intellectual functioning that affects the ability to function independently, communicate, and learn.

metacognition. Use of knowledge to direct comprehension and behavior; involves understanding the demands of the situation and the task and actively employing strategies to plan, monitor, and regulate performance.

metalinguistics. A component of metacognition; use of the ability to analyze, reflect on, and think about language and to apply that ability to understanding a message; involves the use of linguistic knowledge such as phonological awareness skills, familiarity with metaphors and idioms, rules governing language structure and meaning, and ability to use contextual cues to direct comprehension and communication.

modeling. Overtly demonstrating the correct way to produce a word or sentence.

multimodality. Pertaining to the use of several different sensory (or motor) systems together, as in multimodality cuing through visual, auditory, and tactile means.

National Coalition for Auditory Processing Disorders, Inc. (NCAPD). A source of APD-related information and support developed by a parent of a child with an APD and several professionals from throughout the United States.

neonatal intensive care unit (NICU). Hospital placement for newborn infants with significant health concerns who require continuous monitoring and health intervention.

neuroplasticity. The ability of the nervous system to change in response to stimulation or lack thereof; includes reorganization and structural and functional changes in nerves and nerve pathways.

nonverbal learning disability (NVLD). Deficit in nonverbal performance or achievement; may include difficulties with mathematics calculation, visual-spatial skills, art, music, and physical education; verbal, language-based skills are significantly better developed.

oppositional-defiant disorder. A psychiatric disorder involving a recurrent and persistent pattern of hostile behavior toward authority figures; includes behaviors such as arguing with adults, losing control of temper, actively defying rules and regulations, or deliberately annoying others.

orthographic symbols. The written or printed representation of the sounds of a language; dealing with language and spelling.

otitis media. Medical term for middle ear infection, a common illness in children.

otoacoustic emissions (OAEs). A method of assessing inner ear function by recording sound energy emitted by the hair cells of the inner ear via a microphone placed in the external ear canal; frequently used for newborn hearing screening.

otologist. A medical doctor who specializes in the diagnosis and treatment of ear diseases.

Output-Organization Deficit. One of the Bellis/Ferre subtypes of APD; involves difficulty in organizing responses to verbal input; presumably arises from dysfunction in the efferent (outgoing) auditory system and/or the executive control system.

pervasive developmental delay (PDD). General diagnostic term used to refer to severe impairment across many developmental areas; autism falls under the category PDD.

phoneme. The smallest unit of sound in a language that can be discriminated from other sounds; for example, the *k* in *kite* and the *c* in *cool* are considered to be the same phoneme.

phonemic regression. A significant impairment in the ability to discriminate and recognize words and speech sounds that cannot be accounted for by hearing loss; usually seen in the elderly.

phonics. A method of teaching beginning readers to spell and sound out words by associating the speech sound with the letter(s) on the page.

phonological awareness. Awareness of how speech sounds are used in the language, including the ability to manipulate phonemes and to recognize that words are made up of syllables and phonemes.

phonological segmentation. The ability to break up a word into its constituent phonemes (e.g., BLACK = four sounds: B, L, A, CK).

positron-emission tomography (PET). Diagnostic imaging technique in which the patient is given a radioactively labeled compound and the brain's metabolism of that compound is detected and recorded by a computer; assists in determining localization in the brain of various functions.

pragmatics. General term referring to the use of language in specific contexts, including social communication abilities.

presbycusis. Hearing loss resulting from degeneration of inner ear and related structures due to aging.

primary auditory cortex. Portion of the temporal lobe of the brain that is devoted to sound processing; interacts with other brain regions for processing of speech and other acoustic signals.

Prosodic Deficit. One of the Bellis/Ferre subtypes of APD; involves difficulty perceiving tone-of-voice and other cues that signal what the speaker *means* versus what he or she *says*; presumably arises from dysfunction in the non-language-dominant hemisphere of the brain.

prosody. Stress, rhythm, and tone-of-voice aspects of speech that signal shades of meaning and intent.

reauditorization. A strategy in which the listener repeats what was heard to reinforce both the message and the memory trace.

receptive language. General term referring to the ability to receive and understand spoken, written, manual, or other forms of language.

Section 504. Portion of the Rehabilitation Act of 1973 that protects the rights of people with disabilities at work and at school, even if they do not qualify for special education services under IDEA and state criteria.

semantics. A general term used to refer to the meanings of words or groups of words in a language.

sight-word reading. The ability to automatically recognize a word from its unique pattern of letters on the page as opposed to sounding out each letter.

sound blending. The ability to put segregated phonemes together to form a word; e.g., C . . . A . . . T = CAT.

sound-symbol association. Connecting the symbol (or letter) on the page with the sound associated with the letter for the purpose of spelling or reading.

spectrum. The charted bands of waves that make up a light or a sound; in sound, the frequency (or pitch) components of the sound.

speech-language pathologist (SLP). A specialist in the diagnosis and treatment of speech and language disorders; requires at least a master's degree in speech-language pathology for clinical certification by ASHA.

syntax. Term referring to the structure or word order of a language.

temporal lobe. The area of the brain in which the primary and associative auditory areas are found; also involved in memory, learning, and a variety of other abilities.

top-down processing. Term used in information processing theory to refer to the influence of higher-level cognitive or language-related knowledge and skills on sensory perception and interpretation, including auditory processing.

triennial evaluation. The reevaluation of a special education student every three years to confirm continued eligibility for special education and related services and to determine current levels of functioning; federally mandated by IDEA.

universal newborn hearing screening. Hearing screening for all infants shortly after birth (preferably prior to being discharged from the hospital) designed to improve early detection of and intervention for hearing loss; supported by federal funds and mandated in some, but not all, states.

Weschler Intelligence Scale for Children (WISC-III). A standardized test of intellectual functioning that leads to measures of Verbal, Nonverbal, and Full Scale IQ as well as functioning in several cognitive subareas.

word attack. The ability to sound out (or phonologically decode) letters in words for the purpose of reading or spelling; requires both phonological awareness and sound-symbol association abilities.

INDEX